OVERCOME STRESS & ANXIETY NATURALLY

Terry Lemerond
Lynn Wagner, MD

The purpose of this book is to educate. It is not intended to serve as a replacement for professional medical advice. Any use of the information in this book is at the reader's discretion. This book is sold with the understanding that neither the publisher nor the authors have any liability or responsibility for any injury caused or alleged to be caused directly or indirectly by the information contained in this book. While every effort has been made to ensure its accuracy, the book's contents should not be construed as medical advice. To obtain medical advice on your individual health needs, please consult a qualified health care practitioner.

Copyright © 2023 TTN Publishing, LLC, Green Bay, WI

All rights reserved. Except as permitted under the United States Copyright Act of 1976, no part of this publication in any format, electronic or physical, may be reproduced or distributed in any form or by any means, or stored in a database or retrieval system without the prior written permission of the publisher.

Library of Congress Cataloging-in Publication Data is on file with the Library of Congress.

ISBN: 978-1-952507-49-6

Editor: Kathleen Barnes • www.takechargebooks.com
Cover & interior: Gary A. Rosenberg • www.thebookcouple.com

Printed in the United States of America

10 9 8 7 6 5 4 3 2 1

Contents

CHAPTER 1
Stress, Anxiety and the Stress Response, 1

CHAPTER 2
Anxiety and Anxiety Disorders, 13

CHAPTER 3
Chronic Disease: The Stress/Anxiety Connection, 22

CHAPTER 4
Stress, the Adrenals and Blood Sugar, 31

CHAPTER 5
Coping Strategies, 38

CHAPTER 6
Alternative Treatments, 45

CHAPTER 7
The Endocannabinoid System and *Echinacea Angustifolia*, 53

CHAPTER 8
Putting It All Together, 65

CHAPTER 9
Doc to Doc, 69

References, 75

Index, 81

About the Authors, 85

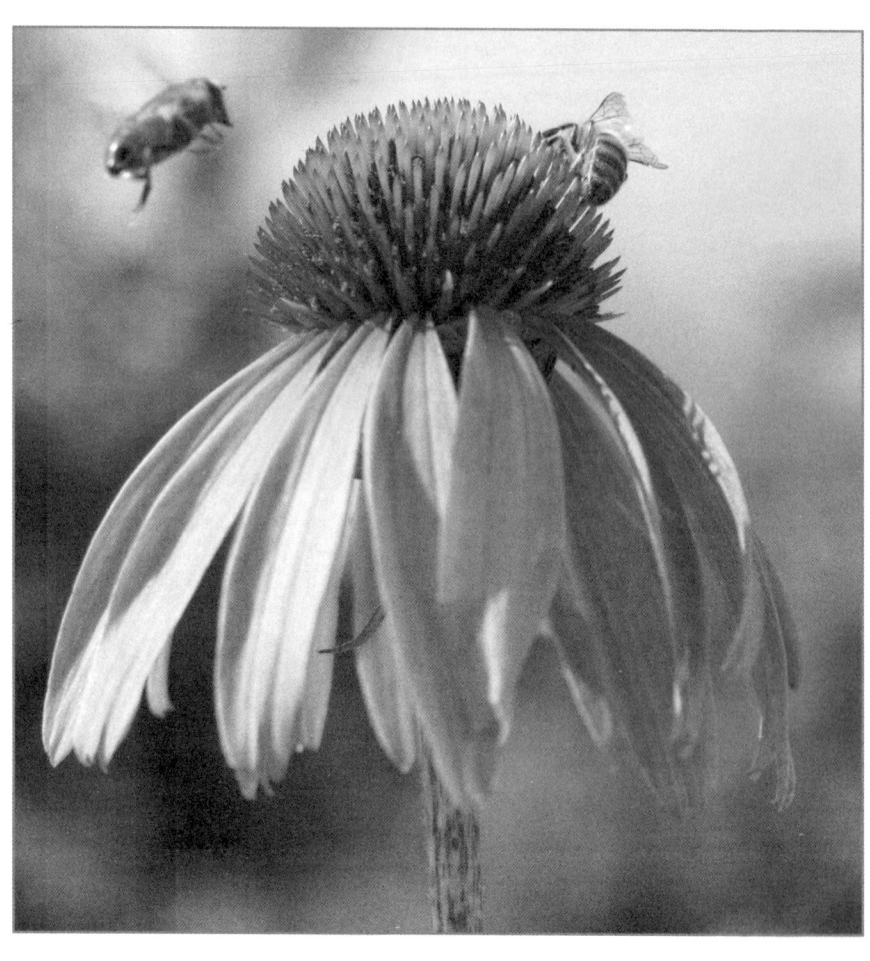

CHAPTER 1

Stress, Anxiety and the Stress Response

Every single one of us experiences stress on a daily basis. Anxiety isn't a stranger to most of us, either. The two actually go hand-in-hand.

You have a conference with your 12-year-old son's teacher, who says he's not completing his classwork. Your spouse's company is about to downsize, and your boss just demanded a report that's going to require a week of evening hours. On top of that, you've had nagging headaches for the past month. And the dog just peed on the floor.

Just reading this litany of stressful woes probably caused you to experience some physiological signs of stress, maybe even anxiety.

So, what do you do? Drink a glass of wine—well, maybe a couple of glasses—and fall into bed exhausted only to wake up at 3 a.m. with your heart pounding and your mind racing:

- What if your spouse's job and income are lost?

- What if your son has a serious problem and is hiding it from you?

- And how can you juggle your own job and family responsibilities?

- What if your ongoing headaches are more serious than first thought?

Over the next week or so, the anxiety spirals out of control and keeps you awake at night, leaves you sleepy at crucial moments of the day and keeps your stomach churning. One time you even wake your spouse for a middle-of-the-night excursion to the ER, since you were convinced you were having a heart attack.

In time, that anxiety may become pathological. Your friends notice you're engaging in obsessive behavior. You can't get your worries out of your mind. The stress sends you into a downward spiral. You visit a doctor who prescribes sleeping pills, antidepressants (oh yeah, anxiety and depression go hand-in-hand, as odd as that may seem—more about that in the next chapter) and anxiety medication—all of which are highly addictive and can cause other serious health problems.

Does this sound familiar? Similar scenarios have become our way of life. Change a detail or two and stress and anxiety have become the norm for most of us.

It's not a healthy norm.

We are fortunate that our bodies have powerful mechanisms to neutralize daily stresses and even the occasional bout of anxiety and still keep us healthy. However, when the stress and anxiety continue, day in and day out, those defense mechanisms break down.

Unrelieved stress and anxiety are the underlying causes of a vast array of health problems, including heart disease and cancer, the two leading causes of death in the Western world.

There is little doubt that chronic stress and anxiety are major contributing factors in many of today's chronic diseases.

New concept in treating anxiety

There are many ways to manage stress. In this book, we'll share with you the ones that offer successful outcomes, including a breakthrough nutrient that is truly exciting because of the positive outcomes we have seen.

Here's a little hint: The often neglected and thinly studied endocannabinoid system of the human body could be on the verge of giving us solutions for anxiety and a number of other health problems. And a familiar plant nutrient provides impressive results with no known side effects.

We've become a sick nation

We're sick and we're not getting any better. With billions and billions of dollars spent every year on chronic diseases, we're really not making any headway towards eliminating the diseases that plague our modern lives.

Cardiovascular disease, including heart attacks, strokes, congestive heart failure and high blood pressure, is as prevalent today as it has been for decades. It's still the leading cause of death in North America, claiming 690,882 lives in 2020, according to the U.S. National Center for Health Statistics.

Cancers, including lung, breast, colon, prostate, colorectal and bladder are quickly challenging heart disease as the leading cause of death in the Western world.

Type 2 diabetes has hit epidemic proportions in both adults and children, and autism and attention deficit and hyperactivity disorder (ADHD) have become common diagnoses in children.

These days, complex chronic diseases like fibromyalgia, chronic fatigue syndrome, myalgic encephalomyelitis (ME), multiple sclerosis and chronic Lyme disease are rarely treated successfully.

So, what's going on? Why can't we get ahead of this disease curve?

We aren't making progress against these chronic conditions because we aren't addressing the underlying issues surrounding them. Even though most health care professionals have a "gut feeling" that anxiety and stress are major culprits in chronic disease, few of us understand why.

Stress and anxiety are the elephants in the living room. While modern medicine tends to look the other way, it's nearly impossible to ignore the connection.

It's time for us to change the way we look at the human body, how it connects to its environment and how our bodies make us what we are.

How do we do that?

It starts on the smallest level.

Here's the most basic primer of the micro level of our bodies and why it's so important to the bigger picture:

Each individual cell and all the 100 trillion cells together in the human body are the drivers of everything that happens to you and your body.

Mitochondria, miniature power plants in the cells, are the drivers of the cells. They produce the energy that runs everything in your body. Each cell may have as many as 1,500 mitochondria that act almost like a digestive system for the cell, taking in nutrients, breaking them down and creating the energy rich molecules that fuel the cell.

Think of your cells like little machines building muscle, bones, hormones, memories, etc. They are reliant on the energy produced by the mitochondria, the electricity that fuels the cells, if you will.

But what if there is not enough electricity or the electrical input is interrupted? The mitochondria don't run very well and, therefore, the cell and the cell systems and organs, and eventually the whole body do not run very well.

External events—like stress and anxiety—have an indirect effect on energy production, and this affects the way your mitochondrial "power plants" function. Numerous studies show that oxidative stress, a direct result of psychological stress and anxiety, impairs the way mitochondria can use the nutrients they receive. When the mitochondria start to malfunction, not enough energy is supplied to cells for all their widely varying functions, resulting in disease.

We also need to change our thinking about the connections between body and mind. This is especially evident when we're talking about anxiety, since much anxiety is the result of a downward thought spiral that starts with worry about something that may or may not happen. When we can rein in the worry process, we can break the vicious cycle. There will be much more about anxiety in Chapter 2.

What is stress?

All of us know stress and most of us have accepted it as part of our everyday lives. Stress can be caused by many different triggers, most of which we perceive as negative: relationships, job pressures, financial pressures, daily traffic and family issues. Stress can also be caused by "good" things like weddings, promotions, the birth of a baby or a move to a new house.

Stress is part of life. The ways each of us as individuals respond to stress can be a determining factor in our overall general health.

Our bodies have incredible mechanisms that are prepared to neutralize these daily stresses and keep us healthy.

Prolonged stress and anxiety can easily spiral out of control, leading to a whole host of other serious health problems.

Stress and Health Problems

Have you ever blamed stress for illnesses? You're not wrong. Unrelieved stress impairs many body functions, including the immune system, so a particularly stressful time can result in acquiring a common cold or the flu—or worse.

No doubt you've heard that a single shocking and stressful event can cause heart attacks and strokes, and, much more often, are the result of long-term stressful Type A lifestyles.

Then it's not much of a leap of logic at all to connect stress to other illnesses.

We'll be delving much more deeply into these connections in the coming chapters, but for now it's important for you to understand that stress and anxiety can contribute to diseases. Of course, we'll also be offering you natural solutions to those destructive effects.

The Zebra and the Lion

When you're under stress, your body engages in a series of physical responses known as the "fight or flight response" stimulated by the sympathetic nervous system that controls involuntary bodily functions like breathing, digestion, wound repair and much more.

The story of the Zebra and the Lion and their encounter is a perfect example of how fight or flight works.

When Zebra catches a whiff of Lion scent, he kicks into panic mode. Clearly, Lion has designs on Zebra as a tasty dinner.

At the moment he recognizes the danger he is in, Zebra needs to make an instant decision: stay and fight the lion (a bad idea if you're a zebra) or run away as fast as he can.

Zebra's body kicks into survival mode. His life is at stake, and he knows it. There is nothing more important to him than survival, so his adrenal glands begin to secrete a hormonal power soup that includes the stress hormones norepinephrine and epinephrine, estrogen, testosterone and cortisol.

The reaction begins with the amygdala, the part of the brain that processes emotional reactions, decision-making and memory.

Zebra's blood pressure skyrockets. A complex series of chemical messengers release a flood of blood sugar and shunt blood from the digestive system, suppresses his immune system, digestion and sex drive, sending all the energy to his limbs so he can run faster. There is nothing more important at that moment than his ability to escape the threat.

After all, if he's dead, what need does Zebra have for digestion or an immune system, much less sex? The importance of energy being shunted away from the gut will become clear when we explore it in depth in Chapter 3.

That hormone flood accelerates heart and lung function, increases blood flow away from the gut (digestive system) to the limbs, liberates glucose and fat stores to give his muscles as much speed and strength as possible and even increases his blood clotting function to prepare for excessive blood loss if he is injured.

His brain can think of nothing but speed, strategy and escape.

We leave our friend Zebra for now, galloping at hyperspeed, the hungry Lion gaining on him. Don't stress, we'll get back to him.

The same things happen to humans when we encounter danger. This is known as the "extreme end" of the stress response.

You've no doubt experienced the fight or flight response yourself.

Think about standing on the edge of a precipice or being in a near-miss car accident and you can even conjure up some of the same body responses:

- hormones are surging through your body
- your heart races
- your pupils become dilated
- you begin to sweat
- you are raring to go and can't stand still.

When you even imagine this scenario, you know without doubt that you're experiencing stress!

Momentary stress isn't really a problem for the human mechanism. It's the long-term unrelieved stress that many of us experience in modern life that opens the door to a host of chronic diseases.

Recognizing the signs of long-term stress is an important component of the stress-reducing regimen: You must acknowledge that a problem exists.

It's important to understand the origin and mechanisms of chronic stress symptoms.

To appreciate the stress response that affects us as humans and all other vertebrates, including our friend, Zebra, indulge me for a few paragraphs to consider the "general adaptation syndrome (GAS)," first recognized by Hans Selye, the father of modern stress research.

The general adaptation syndrome is broken down into three distinct phases:

1. Alarm

2. Resistance

3. Exhaustion

Alarm

The first response to stress, the alarm reaction is pretty much the same as fight or flight. The hypothalamus, our body's master sensor, recognizes the threat and signals the pituitary, the master gland in the base of the brain, to release ACTH, adrenocorticotropic hormone. ACTH is the alarm bell hormone.

This wakes up the adrenal glands, little almond-shaped glands that sit on top of the kidneys, telling them to release stress hormones, adrenaline and cortisol, so you can get moving one way or another, to fight or to run.

Resistance

Once the alarm phase is over (it's usually short lived), the resistance phase kicks in, allowing the body to continue fighting the stressor.

As the stress continues (maybe it's only that you're late for work because you had a sick child), the body adapts to the stressor and mounts a Herculean effort to reduce the effects of the stressor.

If, for example, our friend Zebra has to run for a long time, he will need more energy because he's exhausted his speed-fueling blood sugar levels. Hormones like cortisol and other corticosteroids secreted by the adrenals play key roles in the "resistance" reaction.

Cortisol for example can help create more glucose by pulling in "storage" (glycogen) from the liver and muscle tissue after blood levels have been depleted by the alarm phase. It can also help keep blood pressure elevated as this continues to help promote blood flow to the arms and legs to make it easier to fight or run.

If you're just late for work and not in a fight for your life, your blood sugar and blood pressure are quite likely spiking as your body tries to deal with the continued stress. You may even have a queasy stomach.

If the resistance stage continues for a prolonged period of time, the reduced digestive function can significantly increase the risk of disease, including many autoimmune diseases, diabetes and possibly even cancer, as we'll explain in Chapter 3.

Exhaustion

Now we find ourselves in the final stage of Selye's general alarm system, the exhaustion stage.

In this phase, the stress has continued for such a long time that the body's resistance to the stress has deteriorated, and it may break down completely.

The prolonged need to shunt blood away from the gut leads to a breakdown of the gut lining, literally opening the body to a well-researched variety of chronic diseases that may not, at first glance, seem to be linked.

This places tremendous strain on many organ systems, including the heart, blood vessels, adrenals and immune system. Exhaustion can lead to heart attacks and strokes, among other health challenges.

But there's a big difference between us as humans and our friend, Zebra. Zebra has a real threat to his life. His response is quite literally a life-or-death fight.

Most of us aren't being chased by lions or robbers or murderers (I hope). We aren't literally fighting for our lives every day, but our bodies respond on a daily basis as if we are in a battle for survival.

And for Zebra, if he escapes from Lion (I won't give away the ending of the story), he'll need some serious down time to let his systems rebalance before his next adventure.

In today's fast-moving world, we are constantly being bombarded by a huge number of stressors. It's impossible to escape them and the pressure is always on. We rarely, if ever, take any down time—and that leads to peril.

STRESSORS

Do you recognize the stressors in your life? Some are obvious, some may not be. Here are a few that might spark some response in you.

- Health concerns
- Financial worries
- Relationship problems
- Worries about children
- 24-hour news
- Discrimination
- Crime
- Medical bills
- Disconnected family
- Childcare
- Internet predators
- Violence/drugs in school
- Plane crashes
- Food safety
- Terrorist attacks
- No down time
- Personal conflicts
- Loss of a loved one
- Family dynamics
- End of a relationship
- Negative self-talk
- Catastrophizing
- Perfectionism
- Crowds
- Noise
- Sharing space
- Grief
- Rape
- War
- Weddings
- Moving
- Betrayal
- Boredom
- Criticism
- Embarrassment
- Jealousy
- Shame
- Uncertainty
- Medications
- Job change
- Travel

These worries can be overwhelming. These, and a thousand other stressors are the warning signs. If you are like Zebra and keep running away from the figurative Lion forever, the chronic stress cycle sets in and chronic disease is almost always the result.

Are you having gastrointestinal problems, headaches, insomnia, unidentified pain or just feeling blue? You're on the first rung of that downward ladder of relentless stress.

THE PRICE OF STRESS

Here's just a short list of diseases that have been scientifically proven to be connected to stress. Some of them may seem a little strange, but in the coming chapters, you'll understand how such seemingly wide-ranging problems can come from unrelieved stress.

- Asthma
- Heart disease
- Common cold
- Chronic fatigue
- Depression
- Diabetes
- Fibromyalgia
- Headaches
- Hypertension
- Irritable bowel syndrome
- Psoriasis
- Rheumatoid arthritis
- Ulcerative colitis
- Ulcers

The good news is that you can still climb back up that ladder of unrelieved stress with just a few simple steps and some of nature's most effective medicines. Stay with me.

Anxiety

What's the difference between stress and anxiety?

Stress is day-to-day life. It's caused by *existing* stress factors. In the case of Zebra, stress is caused by Lion who wants to make him dinner.

Stress is our response to the threat. Anxiety is a reaction to the stress after the threat is gone. So, when we experience stress, it is often accompanied with feelings of anxiety.

You can bet if our Zebra escapes from Lion, he'll most likely be trembling for hours after his close encounter with death. He will definitely hide in a place that feels as safe as it can be. He may become hypervigilant, startling with every rustle in the brush. He probably won't sleep for a while as the adrenaline keeps surging through his body.

We're sure you're starting to see where this is going. Anxiety is very often the outcome of unrelieved stress.

Nature created stress and anxiety for a purpose: to protect us from potential threats by giving us physiological tools to combat threats and later putting us into a vigilant state of awareness.

For example, if you are walking through the forest and hear the growling of a bear, the anxiety you feel makes you cautious and keeps you from confronting the bear. This can protect you from a possible danger, so anxiety is doing its job!

Unfortunately, for tens of millions of people, anxiety can occur for no apparent reason. There are no threats, just feelings of uneasiness that create all sorts of agonizing symptoms.

Anxiety can last for moments, hours, days and sometimes even years. When anxiety becomes so entrenched, as in the cases of soldiers who have served in combat zones, it interferes with the ability to function and live a productive life.

In the coming chapters, we'll be examining the effects of long-term stress and how the compromised gut literally opens the door to chronic disease.

Oh—and we know you were wondering if our friend Zebra escaped the Lion. OK—since we're so closely identified with Zebra's heroic efforts to survive, we'll say that Zebra survives and Lion will have to go hungry for a day or two until he finds a less speedy zebra.

CHAPTER 2

Anxiety and Anxiety Disorders

Anxiousness is normal. When it begins to interfere with our daily lives, it becomes a problem.

Anxiety is often defined as "an unpleasant emotional state ranging from mild unease to intense fear." It includes both the emotional and physical feelings we might go through when we are concerned or nervous about something. Anxiety is different from fear, in that fear usually responds to an actual event, while anxiety, in most cases, usually lacks an obvious cause.

Although, some anxiety can be classified as normal and, in some cases, essential, high levels of anxiety contribute to the same health problems as long-term stress.

Most of us know what it feels like to be anxious. All of us can probably remember at least a few times when we've been nervous about something. Perhaps it was just before going to a job interview, the night before writing an entrance exam, moving through a dark alley or walking down the aisle with a future spouse. The feelings in all these circumstances are usually worry, muscle tension, fear, doubts and many more; they are both physical and psychological and the experience is seldom an enjoyable one.

Interestingly, anxiety has its own set of symptoms. Some are physical—like heart palpitations, tightness in the chest, hyperventilation, muscle tension, headaches, excessive sweating, dry mouth, dizziness and even digestive issues. Other symptoms are emotional, like feelings of dread, constantly being on the alert for signs of danger, trouble concentrating, irritability and more.

If you stop to think about it, being anxious during many situations is normal. In some cases, it could actually save your life.

Anxiety is closely linked to our normal biological response to threats, the "fight or flight" response outlined in Chapter 1.

In general, during a period of anxiety, you will experience both physical and psychological symptoms for a short while or till the event has passed—the job interview is over or the performance in front of an audience has passed. Then things usually go back to normal.

I say "usually" go back to normal, because anxiety can become problematic when the feelings become intense, when anxiety continues long after the situation has passed and when the anxiety begins to interfere with daily functioning.

Anxiety disorders affect 40 million Americans age 18 and older. That's 18% of the population. They cost the U.S. over $42 billion a year, almost one-third of the nation's mental health costs.

This high toll underscores the urgency of better understanding anxiety and coming up with more creative solutions for the problem.

Anxiety is normal

As difficult and annoying as anxiety can be, it actually serves an important purpose. All of us have pre-wired (innate) responses to external stimuli, put in place to actually protect us from threats and dangers. These innate responses also allow us to better deal with events occurring in our daily lives.

For example, most people will feel anxious when they give a speech to a large audience for the first time. This anxiety actually serves a purpose: it makes you focus on the speech and makes you want to review and practice the speech over and over again to ensure it flows smoothly. In the end, the initial anxiety allowed you to perform better.

Anxiety also serves to protect you from real dangers, or at least make you more alert to them. Maybe you like to hike far away from the beaten path. You know you could encounter bears, poisonous snakes and even mountain lions. You know they could be around, and you may even see warning signs.

So, you protect yourselves and your fellow hikers by being alert, by not carrying food that would attract bears. You watch for movement in the trees and undergrowth. You might make noise, knowing that, as much as you'd like to avoid meeting them, most of these animals would rather avoid an encounter with you, too. This is a wise response to a real threat.

Again, in this example, anxiety does its job in attempting to protect us from a possible bear encounter. We become more alert to the danger, we are actually moving into a fight or flight response just with the thought of a possible encounter.

We're all wired a little differently and this is also true when it comes to anxiety responses. For example, some people might get anxious over a telephone bill payment and have little to no anxiety about the bear in the forest. We all have pre-wired startle responses, but we also develop responses through various life experiences.

If you nearly drowned as a child, you might have a strong startle response to being in a boat or even thinking about being in a boat.

Or an example for more everyday life, if at some time, your telephone was cut off due to late payment, and the phone plays a big part in your life, you may now have developed a startle response to telephone bills. This anxiety helps protect you from experiencing the stress of losing the ability to talk to others (an important aspect of your life).

When anxiety is not normal

Anxiety is response to a real threat—even if it's just a job interview or giving a speech, much less our friend Zebra and his encounter with Lion—is a normal response. But sometime anxiety persists for days, months, even years. It is often a less-than-rational reaction, perhaps a fear of monsters under the bed or a phobia about spiders. When anxiety becomes persistent, overwhelming and interferes with your daily activities, then you may have a problem and you certainly need to seek medical attention.

There are a number of different types of anxiety disorders, so let's take a little time and review according to the medical classifications.

Here are the most common anxiety disorders, according to the current medical classification system:

Generalized Anxiety Disorder (GAD): Generalized anxiety disorder, affecting 6.8 million adults, is characterized by persistent, excessive, and unrealistic worry and tension about everyday things. These symptoms occur even if there is little or nothing to incite the anxiety. Women are twice as likely to experience GAD than men.

Panic Disorder/Panic Attacks: Individuals with this condition experience feelings of terror out of the blue, repeatedly without warning. Panic attacks sometimes occur even during sleep and are accompanied with chest pain, sweating, heart palpitations and a feeling of choking. Many people often visit the emergency ward because the symptoms often are mistaken for a heart attack. Six million Americans, two-thirds of them women, suffer from this type of anxiety that is closely linked to depression. (More on that coming up.)

Social Anxiety Disorder: More than 15 million Americans suffer from social anxiety disorder in which people feel overwhelming worry and self-consciousness about daily social situations. Their fear of being judged and scrutinized by other people in social or performance situations becomes debilitating. Individuals with this type of anxiety often have limited relationships and are isolated. A recent study showed that more than a third of people with social anxiety disorder experienced symptoms for ten years or more before seeking medical help.

Specific Phobias: This anxiety disorder also affects huge numbers of Americans—19 million at last count. These phobias typically begin in childhood and are defined as strong irrational fears of something that has little or no real danger. Those who suffer from phobias have intense fears of a specific object or situation, for example, high bridges, new places, blood, certain animals, climbing a ladder, flying, being in an enclosed space or in a very open space. Patients with phobias would go to great lengths to avoid being placed in these types of situations.

Obsessive-compulsive Disorder (OCD): Most of us have heard the term obsessive-compulsive or even used it to describe people we know. This diagnosis is given when an individual's anxiety leads them to experience both obsessive and compulsive behaviors. Obsessions are unwanted and intrusive thoughts that come in the form of images, urges or doubts appearing repeatedly in the mind. Compulsions on the other hand are ritualistic behaviors and routines; like washing hands over and over again or counting steps. People with OCD spend a significant amount of time performing pointless tasks and focusing in on obsessive thoughts. This obviously interferes with all aspects of a person's daily life. More than 2 million people suffer from OCD, most of them women.

Post-Traumatic Stress Disorder (PTSD): We've probably heard more about PTSD than most other anxiety disorders because of its prevalence and its connection to returning war veterans. It's estimated that 7.8% of the American population will have PTSD at some point in their lives. While PTSD is generally linked to witnessing or experiencing a traumatic event, we know that PTSD can result from far distant events, including childhood sexual abuse. People with PTSD often have flashbacks or nightmares about their trauma and feel like they are re-living the experience. The anxiety is as intense as the actual event that occurred in their past. Women are twice as likely to develop PTSD as men.

How are anxiety disorders diagnosed?

There are no lab tests to diagnose anxiety disorders, so the only way a healthcare practitioner can diagnose an anxiety disorder is based on the patient's narrative, medical history, elimination of other medical conditions, a physical exam and expert opinion.

In most cases, if the physician has ruled out all other possible causes, the patient will probably be referred to a psychiatrist, psychologist or other specialized health professional able to diagnose anxiety type illnesses.

Signs and symptoms of anxiety disorder

Anxiety has numerous symptoms that are usually short lived. When they last longer than expected, these symptoms can become chronic and lead to anxiety disorders.

Anxiety often manifests with symptoms that originate in the chest, including heart palpitations, sharp pains around the heart, chest tightness and hyperventilating. This is why many people experiencing acute (short-term) anxiety think they are having a heart attack and often end up in the emergency room where tests usually rule out heart involvement.

Longer-term anxiety can cause sleep problems, cold and sweaty hands or feet, dry mouth, numbness and tingling in the hands and feet, nausea, muscle tension, and dizziness. Digestive disturbances are another common symptom, including urgent need and frequent need to urinate and defecate.

People with anxiety disorders often report their minds are racing; they have a sense of impending doom and a difficult time thinking positive thoughts. They frequently are physically very tense and have a difficult time relaxing.

It's important to note here that anxiety and depression are closely linked. Researchers at the University of Texas at Galveston found that half of the adults who visited a doctor for treatment of anxiety also had depression and vice versa. A Columbia University study confirmed that 89% of people they treated for major depression also had a generalized anxiety disorder.

While anxiety and depression are not all the same thing and no one knows exactly why they often occur together, scientists generally agree that malfunctioning brain chemistry is at least one cause of the linkage between these fraternal twins of mood disorders.

Causes of anxiety disorders

Although the exact cause of anxiety disorders is unknown, a combination of brain chemistry and environmental factors are most likely major contributors. Studies have shown that severe and long-term stress can impact nerve cells and their ability to communicate in the brain, thereby contributing to anxiety disorders. There are also some genetic predispositions that may cause anxiety disorders. We'll go into more detail on mechanisms by which anxiety disorders occur in Chapter 8.

Treating Anxiety Disorders

Pharmacological Medications: Conventional physicians will usually use various types of prescription drugs to reduce the symptoms of anxiety. This may include certain types of antidepressants, anti-convulsants, sleep medications and anti-anxiety reducing drugs. The best known is the anti-anxiety drug, Ativan (lorazepam). Doctors are very careful when using this medication, because although it is effective in reducing the symptoms, it's extremely addictive and carries a long list of other side effects, including aggression, memory loss, hallucinations, confusion, suicidal tendencies, tremors and many more.

Coping Strategies: We all have a pattern for coping with stress and anxiety. Some of these coping mechanisms are positive (exercise, relaxation techniques, reaching out to a friend) and others can be destructive (drugs, alcohol, overeating, too much television, etc.). I work closely with my patients to help them make the choices that will replace some of the negative coping strategies with positive ways of dealing with stress and anxiety.

Dietary and lifestyle changes: There is little doubt that making dietary and lifestyle changes will improve your overall health and are also effective coping strategies to manage stress and anxiety. Eating healthy foods, getting a good night sleep, taking the proper dietary supplements and exercise are all steps in the right direction. A healthy and fully functional body has a greater chance of dealing with daily stress and anxiety than a not so healthy body.

Herbal/Nutritional Therapies: It's important to use the best quality and most effective natural supplements with supportive clinical research. Too many times people take products off the shelf that offer little in the way of supportive scientific research and clinical benefits.

Dr. Lynn has made it an essential part of her practice to identify scientifically researched nutraceuticals, observe their clinical effects and share that knowledge with her patients and other physicians. She does not recommend a product unless she has used it on dozens of patients and seen measurable outcomes.

Dr. Lynn has noticed that many of her patients are more interested in alternative therapies then in pharmacological interventions. If there is a more holistic approach to the intervention, eight out of ten patients would rather take the "natural route." We will take a deeper dive into clinically proven alternatives in Chapters 6 and 8.

In the coming chapters, we'll be sharing with you supportive nutritional ingredients that can help with stress and anxiety. There is a particular herbal ingredient that is quite exciting and is giving stunning results with patients with long-term stress and anxiety disorders without any side effects.

ANXIETY AND ANXIETY DISORDERS

WHAT YOU NEED TO KNOW

- Anxiety is a natural response to a threat or a perceived threat, much like the natural fight or flight response to stress.
- Long-term anxiety to a real threat or an imagined threat can become an anxiety disorder.
- Depression and anxiety often go hand in hand.
- There are lifestyle strategies, including diet and nutrition, and natural herbal supplements without side effects that can help cope with anxiety.

ANXIOUS?

This simple questionnaire will help you determine if anxiety is a serious health problem for you. Please rate each question on a 1 to 4 scale:

1. Not at all
2. Several days in the past two weeks
3. More than half the days in the past two weeks
4. Nearly every day

Feeling nervous, anxious or on edge   _____

Not being able to stop or control worrying   _____

Worrying too much about different things   _____

Trouble relaxing   _____

Being so restless it's hard to sit still   _____

Becoming easily annoyed or irritable   _____

Feeling afraid as if something awful might happen   _____

Your score: _____

If your score is 10 or more, you are most likely suffering from moderate to severe anxiety and should seek professional help.

CHAPTER 3

Chronic Disease: The Stress/Anxiety Connection

There's no question that stress and anxiety can have negative health consequences.

Hundreds, if not thousands of published studies detail the risk of chronic disease like heart disease, diabetes, obesity and even cancer from long-term stress.

Anxiety has also been widely proven to lead to gastrointestinal disorders and chronic obstructive pulmonary disorders (COPD). Women diagnosed with anxiety disorders are 59% more likely to have a heart attack and 31% more likely to die of heart attacks than healthy women. People with anxiety disorders are also much more susceptible to ulcers, arthritis, asthma, diabetes and heart disease.

The relationship between stress and illness is complicated. Among the many variables is your lifestyle, as you will see in Chapter 5. Your ability as an individual to cope with stress, your personality traits (extroverts with a high level of conscientiousness have the best ability to find solutions to stress and anxiety) and your genetic predisposition to anxiety and depression can all impact your abilities to cope with stress and neutralize its physical impact.

Our Starting Point

Let's get to the root of the matter: Chronic stress has a significant effect on the immune system. That's the source of this multitude of physical problems that long-term stress and anxiety can cause.

Among its many effects, stress can have an impact on stomach acid concentration. Who hasn't had that queasy-in-the-belly feeling when you've had a near-miss car accident, or you have to give someone bad news?

Now here's something you may not know: That acid concentration in the stomach can contribute to the build-up of plaque in the artery walls leading to heart disease, can be a factor in Crohn's disease, ulcerative colitis and even the development of cancer by suppressing natural killer cells' activity. That gives us just an inkling of how stress and anxiety can have deep and dramatic effects on the whole organism.

Whoa! How do all of these connect? Stay with us.

Gut feelings

In order to understand how chronic stress and anxiety can create so many problems, we're offering a quick primer on the gastrointestinal tract. We'll call it the "gut" for simplicity.

Scientists are now figuring out what Hippocrates—the father of medicine—figured out over 3,000 years ago, when he proclaimed, "Health begins in the gut."

What he was saying is that there cannot be health without a healthy gut.

The gut is the seat of the immune system in the human body.

The past decade or so, much research has substantiated what Hippocrates said, primarily because of the high level of interest in probiotics. We have learned about the microbiome, the collection of microbes or microorganisms inhabiting the gut and creating a kind of mini-ecosystem. Scientists are now churning out thousands of published papers every year on the association between the microbiome and overall general health.

Finally, modern medicine is catching up with Hippocrates and many other gifted healers who have recognized this relationship for millennia, creating a new understanding about how important the gut is to overall health.

Some Background

Today we know that the gut is not only a place of digestion where nutrients are absorbed and wastes eliminated, but also a place where other critically important functions take place. These are functions we wouldn't necessarily associate with the gut, yet they are functions vitally important to the health of the human body.

THE GUT FACTS

Nearly 80% of our immune system is located in the gut.

Let's back up for just a moment. Our bodies are packed with antibodies, proteins that neutralize harmful bacteria and viruses. IgG or immunoglobulin G is the most abundant antibody in the human body, making up 80% of all the antibodies in our system.

Most important for our purposes here, 100% of all IgG is made in the gut. Based on this fact alone, we can say that 80% of our immune system comes from the gut. Are you following the math?

Here's one easy link: Studies show that people under stress are far more likely to have viral infections like colds and flu.

> **The gut is the seat of the immune system in the human body.**

Second, if you think about which part of the human body has the most exposure to the external environment, the gut wins hands down. The gastrointestinal tract has about 430 square feet of surface area, so anything from the outside world has extensive contact with the gut than any other place in our body. It's basically an open system—from the mouth straight down the throat and esophagus, to the stomach to the gut. Think of what you swallow every day, intentionally or not.

Think about this, too: If you were to protect your house from burglars, where would you put the guards? You would place them in the main entry points, the front and back doors!

In the human body, the intelligent immune system would do the same: It places its guards in the main entry point, the gut. So now you can easily see why the immune system is located in the gut.

There are as many neurotransmitters produced in the gut as there are in the brain.

Neurotransmitters are often thought as "brain chemicals," but this is another physiology myth. The gut produces many neurotransmitters, including 85 to 90% of all serotonin, the "feel good" hormone. Antidepressant prescription drugs called SSRIs tell the body to preserve serotonin (in other words, stop its breakdown thus increasing the brain levels and keeping you feeling good). But some experts say these most commonly prescribed antidepressants are no better than placebos.

Could improving gut function improve serotonin levels, thus helping us feel better about ourselves, relieving depression and helping us sleep? We think so!

There are more than 100 trillion bacteria in your gut

Imagine the magnitude of this number and what these little microorganisms are doing in your gut. Much research is being done on these little critters and what we are learning is nothing short of amazing.

Beneficial bacteria are vital to maintaining immune function, the integrity of the gut lining, controlling pathogenic bacteria and even keeping your brain in functional order.

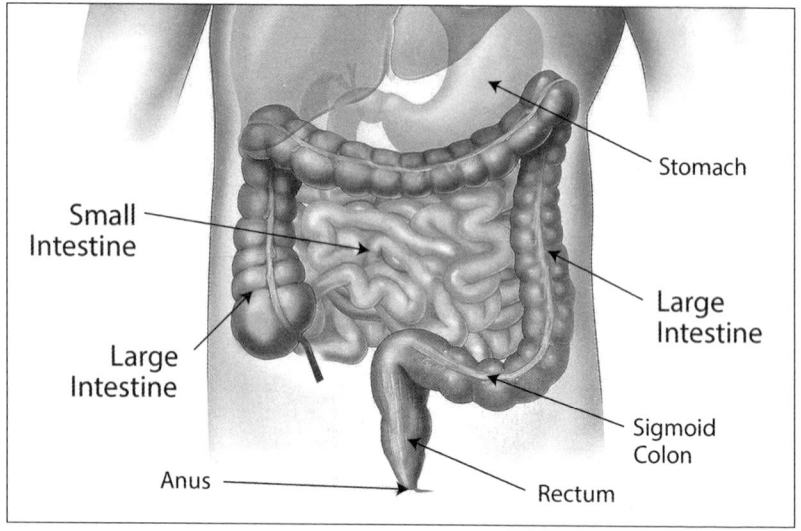

The large and small intestines, also known as the gut.

Recent research into fecal transplantation is giving us new insights and opening up new avenues of treatment for long term gastrointestinal and neurotransmitter problems that could become the norm in the future.

Here's a case that gives us incredible insights into the power of gut bacteria. A 38-year-old woman contracted *C. difficile* (one of the most dreaded gastrointestinal infections, hard to treat and potentially deadly). She had chronic diarrhea and was placed on IV antibiotics. For three months she was hospitalized with no resolution to her infection. She lost nearly 40 pounds and was placed in critical condition. She was at death's door. Then her gastrointestinal specialist went into her husband's gut and isolated bacteria, which he transplanted into her colon. Within three days the *C. difficile* was completely eradicated and the patient made a complete recovery.

It was an incredible observation: Three months of the world's most powerful antibiotics couldn't eradicate *C. difficile*, yet "healthy human gut bacteria" transplanted into the patient's gut did it in three days. This type of treatment has been implemented more than 1,000 times with the same dramatic outcomes. This one case alone offers us an important insight into the power of a healthy gut!

We are merely scratching the surface here, but you may be beginning to understand the importance of a healthy gut and the bacteria it contains.

The one cell paradox

A membrane the thickness of only one single measly little cell separates the gut and the bloodstream. This tiniest of all barriers is all that stands in the way of bacteria, toxins and other harmful compounds from entering the blood stream.

This is a paradox because not only does this one cell lining need to be strong enough to block these compounds from entering the bloodstream, but at the same time it needs to be permeable enough to allow nutrients to get into the blood.

It is this "one cell paradox" that's the fulcrum of many health conditions that lead to increased gut permeability or what in some circles is called "leaky gut." Basically, this means there is a breakdown in that one-cell barrier. Somehow the gatekeeper has gotten confused and is allowing the good guys (nutrients) in as well as the bad guys (pathogens, harmful bacteria and toxins).

Anxiety/Stress and the Gut connection

Now that we have a better understanding of the function of the gut, we can begin to look at the influence that stress and anxiety may have and how this can impact overall health.

The gut is, of course, a place where food gets broken down, nutrients become absorbed and waste products are eliminated. We are well aware this is a simplistic overview.

When we look more closely at this one-cell layer (epithelial layer), we find that an intricate array of proteins known as "tight junctions" firmly hold these epithelial cells together, acting as a gatekeeper to let the good guys through and keep the bad guys in the gut where they belong and where they will eventually be eliminated. The movement of nutrients and other materials through this thin wall is closely monitored and controlled. When this system is functioning properly, everything is good.

However, there are problems that can distract or even disable the gatekeeper.

Have you ever experienced some form of digestive problem? Of course! We all have had an upset stomach, gas, bloating, heartburn, diarrhea or even a bout of constipation.

Just like stress, an occasional bout of digestive distress is nothing to be too concerned about. But when these issues continue over a long term, they can present serious health challenges.

As strange as it may seem, poor gut function is linked to health problems like heart disease, eczema, arthritis, fibromyalgia, chronic fatigue, autoimmune disorders and more. Did you ever imagine that the chronic use of antacids could contribute to developing food allergies and autoimmune diseases?

It all makes sense when you remember the one-cell layer.

You may remember that back in Chapter 1, we introduced the hypothalamus, which controls many bodily functions. When the hypothalamus registers stress, it acts to protect itself. This is when the gut epithelial lining (the one cell separation) can become compromised.

Remember our Zebra and Lion from Chapter 1? Gut compromise is the consequence of the prolonged flight-or-fight response, where the sympathetic response takes blood from the gut (core) and moves it to the peripheral tissues (limbs) in order for the Zebra to run away from the Lion.

In the human body, when we have unrelieved stress and anxiety, the sympathetic response is continuously turned on, creating long term, increased gut permeability, also known as "leaky gut." In simple terms, the gatekeeper goes to sleep on the job and allows all sorts of bad guys through that one-cell layer.

The end result can be autoimmune disease, food intolerances, systemic inflammation with a wide variety of consequences and mitochondrial dysfunction leading to fatigue, sleep disruption, cognitive issues and more.

Stress and anxiety are by far the most important contributors to poor gut function.

The leakiness of the gut walls, the breakdown of the one-cell lining can allow different materials to get into blood and create havoc in the body as illustrated below.

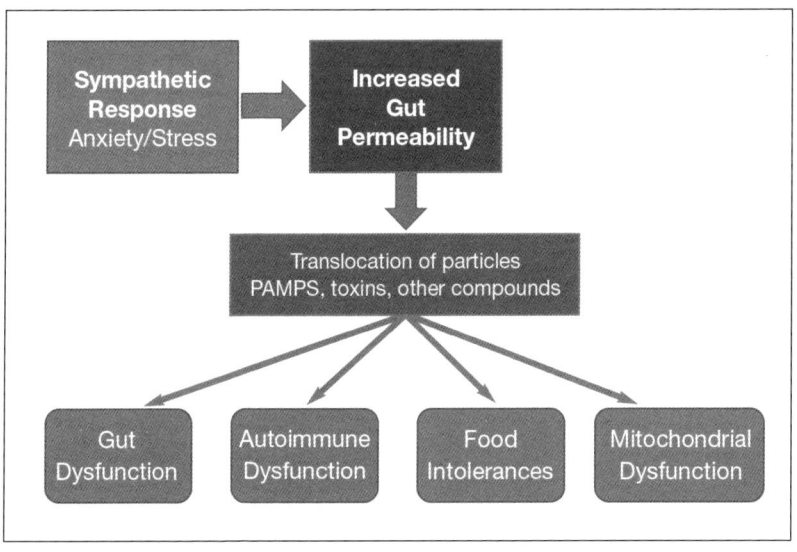

Etiology of Systemic Conditions: Increased gut permeability creating systemic health consequences.

A simplified look

This book wouldn't be complete without a simplified version of "increased gut permeability" and how it relates to systemic health conditions.

If you're confused about how a "leaky" gut could lead to systemic dysfunctions, think about the roof of your house. The roof on your house is your gut lining (one cell thick) and inside your house are items analogous to parts of your body. The sofa, for example, is your skin, the hinges on the doors are your joints, the furnace is your lungs, the television is your brains and so on. Now, imagine if you had holes in your roof during the rainy season. Depending where the holes are, the water would fall on different items around the house.

If it fell on the sofa, it would create mold, that would be analogous to increased gut permeability leading to eczema on our skin. If it fell on the door hinges, they would rust, that would be analogous to increased gut permeability leading to arthritis. And if the water would land on the furnace, that would be analogous to increased gut permeability leading to asthma.

Anybody who has ever had a leaky roof also knows that the leak may travel for some distance, affecting a distant location in the house, or in the body in this analogy.

This can give you a mental picture how a leaky gut is similar to a leaky roof and can inflict seemingly widely separate dysfunctions on the human body.

Stress and anxiety trigger this dysfunction. Therefore, it stands to reason, that in treating gut dysfunction, your health care professional must consider stress and anxiety as key contributing factors and, therefore, relieving stress and anxiety must be paramount in any treatment plan.

CHAPTER 4

Stress, the Adrenals and Blood Sugar

Two grape-sized glands that sit just on top of your kidneys have a profound effect on just about every aspect of your life.

The adrenal glands produce hormones that you can't live without, including adrenaline and the natural steroids aldosterone and cortisol, which are intimately connected to the fight or flight response. They also help your body control blood sugars, break down protein and fat, regulate blood pressure and your body's balance of salt and water, heart rate, levels of minerals in the blood, maintain pregnancy and produce sex hormones.

You can see where we're going here: Prolonged stress and anxiety put a continuous strain on the adrenal glands, eventually causing them to weaken, stumble in their function to produce those essential hormones and eventually to become exhausted.

When your adrenals are fatigued, your entire body is fatigued.

People with adrenal fatigue often complain of feeling overstressed, anxious, overwhelmed and depressed.

Adrenal dysfunction

You remember our friends Zebra and Lion from Chapter 1? Zebra went through the entire stress response preparing to run for his life. His body was flooded with the stress hormones cortisol and adrenaline.

SIGNS OF ADRENAL FATIGUE

1. Trouble waking up in the morning.
2. Cravings, especially for salty foods. Eating salt can actually help improve the situation.
3. Being awake and alert in the evening hours, after 6 p.m.
4. Feeling dizzy when you stand up quickly because your blood pressure is low.
5. Increased allergies.
6. Poor memory.
7. Muscle and bone loss, muscle weakness.
8. Low tolerance for daily stressors.
9. You get sick easily because your immune system is compromised (and you most likely have leaky gut).
10. Blood sugar fluctuations, perhaps even pre-diabetes or Type 2 diabetes.

The adrenals also ensured that his blood sugars were increased for that burst of energy he needed to power his flight for his life.

But when the stress is prolonged, chronic problems almost inevitably arise, leading to adrenal fatigue characterized by blood sugar swings and difficulty regulating blood sugars as well as depression, insomnia, and constant stress.

When adrenal function is disturbed, it changes the way you respond to stress. Constant demand on the adrenals wears them down, leading to adrenal fatigue or adrenal exhaustion.

James Wilson, author of *Adrenal Fatigue: The 21st Century Stress Solution*, estimates that 80% of us will suffer from adrenal fatigue at some time in our lives, yet the condition remains undiagnosed for most sufferers.

It's worth noting here that conventional medicine rejects the idea of adrenal fatigue, almost universally, and some call it a medical myth with no basis in science. Yet the recommended treatment for unrelieved stress is almost exactly what we are recommending in this chapter: stress management, exercise, blood sugar control, sleep hygiene. Call it what you like. A horse (or zebra) of any color is still a horse.

People with adrenal exhaustion are stressed out, tired, prone to allergies, while someone with excessive adrenal activity is likely to have high blood pressure, depression and elevated blood sugar and cholesterol levels.

When we talk about excessive adrenal activity, we're talking about a person who is in "high alert" stress mode. What happens here is that loads of cortisol are injected into the blood by the adrenal glands? The cortisol pulls water into the circulation in order to elevate blood pressure so the zebra can run faster.

Also, the cortisol is going to extract glycogen (a stored form of sugar) from the liver and muscle tissue in order to increase blood sugar for the body's increased needs. Cholesterol will also have to go up because guess how cortisol is made? You got it, from cholesterol. On the short term, this is all fine. On the long term, it means trouble.

WHAT CAUSES ADRENAL FATIGUE/ EXHAUSTION?

- Unrelieved stress
- Anger, fear, anxiety, guilt
- Physical, mental and emotional strain
- Too much exercise
- Too little sleep
- Temperature fluctuations
- Chronic illness or chronic inflammation
- Toxic exposure
- Physical trauma, especially from surgery or injury
- Blood sugar roller coaster

So how is all this related to stress and anxiety?

The body senses all of the above as stress. For example, when your sugar levels drop, the hypothalamus (body sensor in the brain) immediately sends signals to the adrenal glands to secrete cortisol and adrenaline to try to raise your blood sugar.

Elevated cortisol levels are not only associated with increased feelings of stress, but also loss of appetite control, cravings for sugar, and weight gain. It can also be a major factor in reducing your ability to cope with stress.

The negative effects of excess cortisol

When your body is in a constant state of stress and anxiety, your adrenals are in overdrive producing hormones like cortisol, most often in a fruitless effort to counteract the stress.

A case in point here is the prescription drug, a corticosteroid called prednisone, an artificial form of cortisol, helps us see the effects of excess cortisol on our bodies. Prednisone is used primarily to treat allergies and inflammatory issues like asthma and rheumatoid arthritis.

This disruption of the body's normal defense functions of the white blood cells is great at stopping the inflammatory response, but it essentially cripples the immune system.

Common side effects of long-term prednisone use at higher dosage levels include depression, insomnia, mood swings, personality changes, psychotic behavior, high blood pressure, diabetes, peptic ulcers, acne, excessive facial hair in women, muscle cramps and weakness, thinning and weakening of the skin, osteoporosis and susceptibility to the formation of blood clots.

Here's the rub: long-term unrelieved stress causes ALL of the side effects that prednisone causes because stress triggers the adrenals to produce too much cortisol.

Cortisol excess is almost always associated with weight gain.

Not only does cortisol signal the brain to eat more, it signals the body to hold onto fat, especially dangerous abdominal fat.

What can you do?

Adrenal stress leading to fatigue and exhaustion is at the core of complex diseases. Commonly, people with impaired adrenal function have low blood pressure, low blood sugar or blood sugar swings, a feeling of dizziness when going from lying to standing position, heart palpitations and difficulty sleeping.

This is where our special botanical that supports healthy adrenal function can give you improved energy levels and also help your adrenals to function better and, hopefully, to heal.

Interestingly, many people think that taking an adrenal support formula will quickly change their fortunes and improve some of their symptoms. It takes weeks or even months to jump start the adrenals. If you have a high stress lifestyle, you may require lifelong supplementation to keep your adrenals functioning optimally.

Protein and adrenal support

Protein is the next key to adrenal health.

Most people think of muscle building when they think of protein supplements. It's true that those bulging muscle folks do use protein supplements, but protein has benefits for everybody, especially people who are stressed and anxious.

It may seem surprising in today's world, but many people just aren't getting the amount of protein they need. The average person is getting a little protein in the morning, a moderate amount at lunch and an adequate amount at dinner. That leaves them with a protein shortfall for the day and leaves their adrenals under-supported.

Dr. Loren Cordain, Professor, Department of Health & Exercise Science, Colorado State University, author of *The Paleo Diet*, believes a high protein diet of 20–40% protein should be the norm.

The average protein intake in the US is about 98 grams a day, but Cordain says (somewhat controversially) this is not enough. He recommends a daily protein intake for the average American male of 125–186 grams of protein a day, and for the average American female 89 to 133 grams a day.

Cordain recommends that increased protein intake should come primarily from lean animal protein, based on the diet our hunter-gatherer ancestors ate—meat, seafood, fruits, vegetables, and nuts.

If you're suffering from adrenal fatigue, raising your protein intake can provide adrenal support and, in time, relief from chronic stress.

Adrenal support nutrients

When you have adequate protein intake, a good adrenal support formula can help. This combination of ingredients should be taken either in the morning or at lunchtime.

Here are some of the useful ingredients you should be looking for.

Nutrients

Adrenal Extracts: Look for a formula that has freeze-dried adrenal extracts. These compounds are usually made from animal adrenal glands. If you want to build muscle, one of the best ways of doing it is to consume animal muscle: for example, by eating a steak. Although there are no clinical studies on adrenal extract, in our experience, they do work.

Look for capsules providing about 200–250 mg per day.

Vitamin B5 (Pantothenic Acid) and Vitamin B6 (pyridoxal-5-phosphate): Both these B-vitamins are essential for the production of all adrenal hormones, including cortisol.

Look for capsules providing 50 mg of Vitamin B5 and 5 mg of Vitamin B6 of the active pyridoxal-5-phosphate per day.

L-tyrosine: This amino acid is a precursor of epinephrine and norepinephrine, two well-known adrenal hormones involved in the "fight or flight response."

Look for capsules containing 200–225 mg of L-tyrosine per day.

DHEA (dehydroepiandrosterone): This hormone is naturally produced by adrenals, and insufficient adrenal function means you most likely aren't producing enough DHEA. It is worth using to help re-build optimal adrenal function.

Men should take 25–50 mg of DHEA per day and women should take 15–25 mg.

Pregnenolone: This "mother of all hormones" is produced in the adrenal glands. Aldosterone, cortisol, progesterone, DHEA are all produced from this base hormone, pregnenolone. This hormone has no known serious side effects.

Look for a product that offers 15 mg per day.

Generally speaking, there really hasn't been a natural go-to compound that consistently gives anxiety sufferers the fast relief they need. Until now.

Stay tuned. In Chapter 7, we'll be giving you the details of a breakthrough supplement that gives fast relief for stress and anxiety that works through a newly recognized physiological system known as the "endocannabinoid system."

CHAPTER 5

Coping Strategies

So—what happens to your stress levels when you're sitting on a beach? Taking a walk with a friend? Taking a long bath? Listening to a symphony?

You are well aware that you relax a little—or a lot—when you engage in favorite activities. We've all experienced it, so we all know that we can take control of our stress and anxiety levels and tone them down, maybe even completely de-stress and stop the anxiety spiral. You've no doubt discovered your own de-stressors.

Remembering that we do have control and we can take control is probably most difficult when we're in the midst of a crisis.

It's important to remember that unrelenting stress can also spark the seeds of debilitating anxiety, so using these tools to break the stress cycle can prevent anxiety from taking over.

Here is a list of time-honored coping skills that may help. Feel free to add your own!

Cognitive behavior therapy (CBT)

This is a deeply researched and scientifically validated form of psychotherapy that is literally intended to change the way you think. It's been found to be very successful in treating anxiety disorders, which, as you will recall from Chapter 3, come from worry about what might happen rather than focus on actual events.

Research has shown that CBT is effective in treating panic disorder, phobias, social anxiety disorder, generalized anxiety disorder, depression, addiction disorders and others. Some therapists who use CBT think it is better in treating anxiety than pharmaceutical drugs.

In a nutshell, CBT is based on the concept that how you think affects how you feel. In other words, your thoughts directly affect your feelings and your actions. It's not actually the situation that generates the stress, but your feelings about the situation.

For example, if you were bitten by a black dog as a child, in the future, you might become anxious every time you see a black dog. You know it is not logical to think that every black dog you encounter for the rest of your life will bite you. CBT can help you change your negative feelings about the dog, which other people might see as a sweet pet. When you become really adept at CBT, who knows? You might even find yourself with a cute Black Lab puppy!

Here's a simple example from everyday life:

DAY BEFORE BIG EXAM ⟶ THOUGHTS...

- I am not ready for the exam.
- My mind will go blank—I am definitely going to fail.
- Everybody is going to think I am dumb.
- I'll never make it.
- I am just not good at this.

CBT makes people aware of their negative thoughts and their behavioral actions supporting the skewed thoughts. CBT helps people change their way of thinking and behaving, ultimately breaking the vicious cycle of negative thinking and reducing the stress and anxiety.

Of course, you need a well-qualified psychotherapist to help you start to recognize those negative thought patterns and learn how to shift them.

Other ways of coping

Exercise

Exercise is a natural stress buster. It actually causes your body to release chemicals called endorphins that interact with your brain's communications system and reduce your perception of pain, and even trigger a positive feeling in the body similar to that of the powerful pain killer, morphine. This may partly explain why some people become "addicted" to exercise, because they love the feeling of wellbeing it provides. Not to worry, this is a good addiction unless, like anything else, you take it to an extreme.

A half-hour walk or swim every day can provide surprising stress relief. Research shows that as little as 30 minutes of daily exercise like walking at a moderate pace can reduce anxiety levels significantly. Some studies show that exercise is as effective at relieving anxiety as prescription drugs, with no side effects except the side benefit of having a healthier body. One large analysis of many studies found that even a short burst of exercise can break an anxiety event like a panic attack.

Let us just point out here that nature heals. It's one thing to walk on your treadmill for half an hour while watching the news (more about that later) and an entirely different thing when you spend half an hour walking in the woods. Voluminous research shows that being in nature increases feelings of wellbeing, reduces the production of stress hormones, lowers blood pressure, slows heart rate and relieves muscle tension. If you have a choice, choose to exercise outdoors.

Relax

When you are on a beach, walking along the sand, hearing the soothing sounds of the waves and smelling the waters' fresh scent, how do you feel? That's right, you feel relaxed, you feel at ease, your worries seem to disappear for that short time. What you just experienced was the art of relaxation.

There are many ways to relax. Since you can't always walk the beach, practicing other forms of relaxation techniques can go a long way in helping you cope with stress and anxiety.

Meditation, yoga, tai chi, breathing exercises, visualizations, specific focused hobbies that take your mind off daily activities all can bring about a feeling of relaxation. You're forgetting your worries and your mind is detoxifying or taking a break from the busy lifestyle you lead. This allows you to change your focus that ultimately changes your thoughts and thus allows you to relax.

Hypnosis

Hypnosis has been shown to reprogram your brain to break the cycle of stress and anxiety.

An experienced hypnotherapy practitioner will start by asking you to talk about your problem. When hypnotherapy is induced, you will be asked to bypass your critical mind, which breaks the negative thinking patterns with much the same result at CBT. In addition, it allows your brain's natural inclination to find solutions to help resolve the problem and even give you tools to address the problem if it arises again.

Two other associated psychotherapies, EMDR (eye movement desensitization and processing) and EFT (emotional freedom technique) can also have profound effects in repatterning thought processes. Check them out.

Learning How to Breathe

"Ha!" you say. "Of course, I know how to breathe! I would not be alive if I didn't know how to breathe!"

That's true, but most of us don't know how to breathe in the most efficient way, in a way that will relieve stress and anxiety. Deep breathing is the key to deep relaxation.

Have you ever noticed how a baby breathes? With each breath, the baby's abdomen rises and falls because the baby is naturally breathing with its diaphragm, a dome-shaped muscle that separates the chest cavity from the abdominal cavity. That's also the way most adults breathe when we sleep. But somehow, when we're awake, we don't consciously remember to breathe correctly.

When we're awake, most of us breathe in the upper chest, using only about one-third of our lung capacity and not using the diaphragm, designed to draw air into the entire lung. Shallow breathing tends to produce tension and fatigue, and deep breathing tends to reduce stress.

Diaphragmatic breathing, sometimes called yoga breathing, belly breathing or singer's breath, is perhaps the most powerful method of breaking the stress cycle and creating calm energy.

This method of breathing is actually our natural way of breathing, and dramatically changes our bodies and our minds by activating the relaxation centers in the brain.

With everything that's going on in our lives, if we had to remember to breathe, most of us would be dead in an hour or so!

EASY GUIDE TO BELLY BREATHING

Here is a 10-step technique for learning diaphragmatic breathing.

1. Find a comfortable and quiet place to lie down or sit.
2. Place your feet slightly apart. Place one hand on your abdomen near your navel. Place the other hand on your chest.
3. You will be inhaling through your nose and exhaling through your mouth.
4. Concentrate on your breathing. Note which hand is rising and falling with each breath.
5. Gently exhale most of the air in your lungs.
6. Inhale while slowly counting to 4. As you inhale, slightly extend your abdomen, causing it to press outward into your hand about 1 inch. Make sure that you are not moving your chest or shoulders.

7. As you breathe in, imagine the warmed air flowing in. Imagine this warmth flowing to all parts of your body.
8. Pause for 1 second, then slowly exhale to a count of 4. As you exhale, your abdomen should move inward.
9. As the air flows out, imagine all your tension and stress leaving your body.
10. Repeat the process until a sense of deep relaxation is achieved.

Sleep

Sometimes it seems like it's a bit of the chicken and the egg: You can't sleep because you're stressed and you're stressed because you can't sleep. It seems like a can't-win situation.

About 40% of Americans suffer from sleep disorders and most of us have occasional insomnia or daytime sleepiness due to lack of restorative sleep at night.

It's not surprising considering the levels of stress most of us experience even in a "normal" day.

Even with sleep medications, most of us do not find deep, restful sleep. Lack of deep, restful sleep can negatively affect virtually every aspect of our lives and even contribute to the chronic diseases we've covered earlier in this book.

More than 9 million Americans use prescription sleep aids, which have terrible side effects. Uncountable others use over-the-counter sleep medications with varying degrees of success. Millions of others look for a natural route with melatonin, valerian, hops, lavender, chamomile and other botanical sleep aids without side effects. While these natural ways restore sleep, they may not be as effective as you'd like if you are truly suffering from anxiety.

All of the coping strategies we've mentioned in this chapter will help with sleep problems. But stay tuned. There is a powerhouse botanical—echinacea, the familiar herb used to treat colds and flu, newly discovered that, when processed in a specific way, will help restore deep restful sleep and possibly bust the stress-anxiety cycle in minutes.

Lifestyle Habits and Coping Patterns

Your body is always trying to reach physical, emotional and mental balance.

Whether or not you are aware of it, your body has developed its own ways of coping with stress and anxiety, although some of those coping mechanisms might not be healthy on any level. Some of those destructive "stress management" techniques might involve alcohol or drug abuse, or other addictive behaviors.

Some people binge watch TV or never turn off the disturbing news, or obsessively eat junk food, or order unneeded items from the shopping channels. I'm sure you recognize these negative coping strategies, and you may even have engaged in some of them yourself.

The best part of your strategy for stress should be to create your own custom strategies that you know will work for you and help you bust the cycle that can lead to life-altering anxiety. As we discovered early on, the best first step comes from the Alcoholics Anonymous 12 Step Program, but applies to many negative behavior patterns: First, recognize there is a problem.

Finally...

Don't underestimate the innate healing power of the human body and mind. Some of these simple techniques, like a few minutes of deep breathing or a 15-minute walk after work, or a yoga class, can give you the profound stress relief your body and mind crave.

CHAPTER 6

Alternative Treatments

Most of us stressed-out, anxiety-ridden folks of the modern world would rather take naturally based compounds than pharmaceutical drugs.

That's a smart strategy since pharmaceuticals for stress and anxiety have serious side effects and they're highly addictive. Side effects for anxiolytic medications (anti-anxiety drugs like Xanax, Ativan, Valium, etc.) are daunting. They include depression, seizures, sexual dysfunction, headaches, drowsiness, confusion, slurred speech, lack of coordination, difficulty breathing and more.

Yes, we understand that some people become so desperate because of their anxiety that they are willing to do anything to stop it. What if we told you there are some safe and natural alternatives that have NONE of these side effects? More importantly, what if we told you that many of these natural alternatives are validated by solid science? And better yet, there is a unique botanical formulation that can stop a panic attack in minutes. We're pretty sure we've got your attention now.

Let's pause for a very brief explanation how various anti-anxiety prescription drugs work.

Two pharmaceutical bad guys

Most patients with chronic anxiety are prescribed one of two types of anxiety medications: benzodiazepine like Xanax, Librium, etc.

and SSRIs (selective serotonin uptake inhibitors) like Prozac, Zoloft, Paxil and more.

SSRIs are technically antidepressant medications (remember anxiety and depression often go hand-in-hand). They work by sending messages to your brain to reduce the re-uptake and breakdown of serotonin (the feel-good brain chemical, neurotransmitter) thus increasing the levels of this compound. SSRIs do help increase serotonin levels, but they don't really help address the problems of low serotonin production by your brain. The drugs work for some people but don't work for others, for reasons we don't entirely understand.

A study published in the *Journal of the American Medical Association* says that SSRIs are no more effective than a sugar pill and work only in about one-third of people with severe depression who take them, despite the serious side effects. Side effects include headaches, blurred vision, nervousness, agitation, insomnia, diarrhea, nausea, sexual dysfunction and more.

The FDA has approved SSRIs for people with general anxiety disorder and panic disorder, but a recent analysis of all of the studies done of this, the benefits of SSRIs were very small and the risks of serious side effects made them a poor choice, according to researchers.

Yet research shows that these medications are often prescribed. One 2011 study found that 23% of women in their 40s and 50s were using SSRIs and 14% of all white adults. (Statistics show Hispanics and African-Americans are less likely to seek any kind of treatment for depression than Caucasians.)

Benzos—or benzodiazepines—are a class of drugs specifically designed to address anxiety as I mentioned earlier in this chapter.

Benzos such as Xanax, Librium, Ativan, Valium and others work on the central nervous system, on GABA (gamma-amino butyric acid) receptors in the brain that slow down reactions and act to depress overactive responses often found in people with anxiety disorders.

Benzos are moderately effective and fast acting, but they are so highly addictive that it is often recommended they only be taken for short periods of time. They become ineffective over time and require greater dosages for the same result. We've already detailed the side effects of benzos—something all of us would want to avoid.

In addition, there's an additional danger: Both of these types of drugs can mess with your brain chemistry. We simply don't know the long-term results of such chemical interference.

These drugs do not "cure" anxiety disorders. They are usually short-term Band-Aids that create long-term physical problems.

This is why many patients with anxiety disorders and a growing number of doctors are seeking natural alternatives that can give them quick relief without side effects. This is not easy to accomplish, but there is good news.

In Chapter 7, we'll be introducing a unique, natural treatment for stress and anxiety that has supportive scientific evidence to give you relief without side effects.

Background

Two main parts of the brain are responsible for triggering anxiety: the amygdala (the brain's emotional center) and HPA-axis (hypothalamic-pituitary adrenal axis).

The amygdala's primary role is to act as a threat detection system or a central location for the generation of anxiety. It is responsible for the perception of emotions such as anger, sadness and fear as well as controlling of aggression.

Interestingly, the amygdala has a memory function to retain events and experiences so that you can recognize similar events in the future. For example, if you've been stung by a bee, your amygdala would store that event, and next time you see a bee, it would prompt you to be cautious and perhaps even fearful and anxious.

It is believed that anxiety disorders often are the result of some imbalance in the neurotransmitters responsible for the function of the amygdala: sedating GABA, calming dopamine and mood-lifting serotonin. That's why natural products like the ones listed below offer healing to people with long-term and even deep-seated anxiety disorders.

The dietary demons are sugar and caffeine

So, here's the one inescapable conclusion: Diet plays a key role in all things to do with your health. Although you may be wary of dietary directives, your control of your diet has a greater effect on your health in the short and long-term than any other factor in your life.

Will it make it easier to swallow (pun intended) if we give you just two strong dietary admonitions when it comes to stress and anxiety?

There is more than enough evidence to convince us—and it should convince you, too—that eliminating sugar and caffeine from your diet can have a profoundly positive impact on your levels of anxiety and help relieve stress in general.

Sugar

Sugar does not cause anxiety, but it definitely affects your body's "environment" and creates obstacles to your body's self-healing abilities.

The average American consumes about 200 pounds of refined sugar every year. This is the sugar found in soda, sweets, baked goods, candy and the sugar you put in your coffee or tea every morning. It's also the hidden sugar in processed foods and even meats.

It's disguised under many names like dextrose, cane sugar, barley malt, maltose, sucrose and, of course, the most damaging of all: high fructose corn syrup. Sugar is everywhere!

Artificial sweeteners are just as damaging for other reasons. Avoid them, too.

When Dr. Wagner's patients are advised to eliminate or even reduce the amount of sugar they consume, they almost always ask the same question: "Besides contributing to diabetes, why is sugar so bad?"

This is a fair question. Sugar in all its forms causes a cascade of serious health consequences.

Excess sugar in the blood and tissues causes a body process called glycation. In simple terms, this is the ability of sugar to "stick" to things. Think about a can of soda. You drink it and when you pick it up for recycling the next day, it's sticky. That's because sugar almost acts like glue. Inside your body, glycation makes sugar stick to protein and fat molecules in your body causing DNA breakdowns that can have far-reaching impacts on your health.

Long-term exposure of your cells to sugar creates AGES (advanced glycation end substances). These compounds can have numerous major effects on your DNA and other cell structures and expose you to high risk for chronic diseases like diabetes, heart disease, cancer, Alzheimer's disease and more. The effects of AGES are especially in people with diabetes who, even with diabetes medications, frequently develop diabetic complications like heart disease, strokes, diabetic retinopathy (blindness), kidney failure and nerve damage that can lead to amputations.

Caffeine

Here's the second dietary demon: Caffeine contributes directly to stress and anxiety. Have you ever gotten that jittery feeling after two or three cups of strong coffee? That's the caffeine revving you up, in very much the same way your body responds to stress. It's like you're always running away from that Lion and eventually, your body becomes dependent on that lift.

Do you often feel sleepy and need some coffee around 4 p.m. just to make it through the rest of your day? That's because your adrenals are weary and need some stimulation to carry you through.

The prolonged demands on your adrenals can eventually wear them out, as we learned in Chapter 4.

That jittery feeling generated by caffeine impacts your sleep quality, too. For many of us, caffeine stays in the system for 12 hours or more. And, of course, coffee is not the only course of caffeine in our diets. Tea (even green tea) and soft drinks all contain substantial amounts of caffeine, not to speak of those "energy" drinks.

Published research confirms that caffeine causes anxiety in several ways by increasing the stress hormones cortisol and epinephrine, reducing calming GABA neurotransmitters, causing low blood sugar, depleting nutrients and reducing blood flow to the brain.

Now when you combine caffeine and sugar (something commonly done), the outcome is multiplied.

The bottom line: If you are suffering from anxiety and stress, you need to reduce or eliminate the sugar and caffeine in your diet.

We love our coffee, but we're here to tell you, if you are suffering from stress and anxiety, it's not good for you. Decaf may be somewhat better, if you must have your coffee, and stevia is a healthy alternative to sugar and artificial sweeteners.

Natural anxiety relief

Many of us like to relax with a calming cup of tea before bedtime. It may not be a conscious choice, but that chamomile tea is a scientifically validated way to stop the overactive brain cycling and help you get restful sleep.

You may even have used valerian root tincture or hops in your tea, or a lavender essential oil as sleep aids.

Here's an important note about nutraceutical and botanical supplements that you may be considering: Most of them do not work quickly, so they will not be effective in the midst of a panic attack, for instance. They take time to build up in your body, sometimes weeks of daily supplementation, so they are more effective to prevent stress and anxiety than to treat full-blown anxiety disorders.

That said, there is one powerful anti-anxiety herb, a unique formulation of *Echinacea angustifolia*. It works within minutes and in studies has been proven to be safe and effective even in the midst of panic attacks and other acute anxiety problems. In Chapter 7, we'll give you all the details of how and why echinacea has these unique qualities in the plant world.

The right stuff

Not all supplements or their ingredients are created equal. Be cognizant of the brand you choose. What is on the label may or may not reflect the true ingredients in a product and those ingredients may not be scientifically accurate.

The U.S. Food and Drug Administration strictly regulates all prescription drugs, so you know that the blood pressure medication or antibiotic that is prescribed for you is exactly the same every time and that their chemical makeup is identical every time.

Unfortunately, the nutraceutical world doesn't fully work that way. Before we get too sidetracked on what could be the subject of an entire new book, let us say that we fully support the supplement industry, but as is the case in any industry, there are sometimes unscrupulous players. It's impossible to give you information on every single supplement, so we can only suggest that you look for well-reviewed products from trusted manufacturers and those recommended by your health care practitioner.

The manufacturing process can also vary widely between products, and some companies will attempt to use cheap ingredients that are completely ineffective, or worse yet, as adulterated with harmful ingredients.

There are many high-quality brands out there—but it may take a little research on your own to find out which ones are the best. Your doctor will probably know and you can get some good advice from your local health food store and other health care practitioners. It's essential to identify brands that use clinically studied ingredients manufactured in such a way that they actually work.

A final note...

Many of us forget the power of the human body to heal itself. Your body is the most intricate and incredibly sophisticated system ever assembled, far more powerful than any computer. It carries out millions of functions every minute, communicating between the nervous system and your 100 trillion cells around it. Its ability to heal is an astonishing feat that it carries out 24/7 throughout your life, mostly without you giving it a first or second thought.

Each human body really has an inborn ability to heal itself given the right environment.

CHAPTER 7

The Endocannabinoid System and *Echinacea Angustifolia*

If you've read this far, you're probably well informed enough to know that echinacea is a well-researched and proven remedy for colds and flu. That's because it boosts the immune system.

Now, surprising and cutting-edge research gives us *Echinacea angustifolia* as an exciting solution for stress and anxiety disorders.

Just to re-cap information from earlier chapters, we're not talking about the occasional stress over being late to work or the anxiety of having to give a speech. We're talking about the serious health effect of long-term relentless stress that many of us suffer and the anxiety disorders that can make it difficult or impossible to cope with everyday life.

Getting back to echinacea, it's one of the best-known herbal remedies in the world. Then, how can it be that we are just discovering its stress- and anxiety-relieving effects after millennia of use?

First, we've learned that only one species of echinacea has these effects and only if it is grown under controlled conditions and processed using special extraction techniques to isolate the active components that impact anxiety and stress.

Second, you can take all the echinacea you want, but unless it contains the right compounds, in the right amounts to impart anxiolytic (anti-anxiety) effects, it just won't work.

It took a team of European researchers to unlock the secret from echinacea and to produce the right combination.

What makes this formulation different from other echinacea?

The first breakthrough came when researchers at the Hungarian Academy of Sciences found that some of the echinacea plants contained compounds known to influence brain chemistry and greatly reduce anxiety. Researchers then performed additional experiments. Their further exploration revealed that it is not just the species of echinacea that is important, but how the plant is grown and how the key compounds are extracted that determines whether or not the extract will be effective against anxiety. While it might look the same as the lovely purple flowered plant with downturned petals that may grow in your garden, but the way it's grown and harvested makes it very different.

In a comparison test of seven different echinacea extracts, only one—*Echinacea angustifolia* root—had high enough levels of those special compounds associated with anxiety relief. These compounds are able to safely bind to brain receptors that trigger feelings of calm and relaxation.

Once they made this huge discovery, the researchers set about finding ways to extract and concentrate these unusual compounds.

Reduce tension, relieve stress and anxiety

In a series of scientific studies, this specific extract was compared to other anxiety-relieving substances. The results found that it not only met or exceeded their effects, but also did not cause drowsiness, a common side effect of prescription anti-anxiety drugs, or any other side effects.

The anxiety busting formula was then tested in human volunteers who reported experiencing increased stress and tension. A standardized assessment tool was used to measure their feelings of anxiety at the beginning of the study and compared with responses 1, 3, and 7 days after taking the specialized extract. After one day of use, the participants experienced a significant reduction on the anxiety measurement scale, which increased to a 25% reduction by Day 7.

Additional laboratory tests have confirmed that this special extract is free of side effects, even at dosages much higher than recommended for anxiety-reducing effects.

Not only does this echinacea extract deliver on the promise of quick relief for anxiety, it works on the endocannabinoid system—unique body system that has brought science to a new way of treating this debilitating disorder.

Discovery

The human body consists of numerous systems, all of which function in concert much like the instruments in an orchestra. These systems include the nervous system, the lymphatic system, the gastrointestinal system, the cardiovascular system, the endocrine system and so on.

Scientists have discovered a new system in the last two decades, and it's now finally gaining recognition for its importance.

The endocannabinoid system not only contains the largest number of receptors of any system in the human body but also produces compounds that have far-reaching health benefits.

So, OK, what are receptors and why are they so important?

This intricate organization of activating compounds and receptors—think of them as receivers and messengers—holds the keys in helping control anxiety and stress.

Aren't cannabinoids the compounds in cannabis (marijuana) that cause you to mellow out? Absolutely, yes! The terms cannabinoids and endocannabinoid are often used interchangeably.

Cannabinoids induce a state of calm and relaxation, exactly like the effects of marijuana.

But maybe you don't want to use mind-altering substances. That's fine. You can get exactly the same effects from Echinacea without the "high" and without any negative results on tests required by some employers. You get the best of both worlds without any negative effects.

The endocannabinoid system (ECS)

Bear with me for a few paragraphs while we introduce you to the endocannabinoid system (ECS) and how it works.

Like your smart phone, it's an information delivery system. The phone receives the messages from the cell tower and it can then pass on information to other parts of the body as needed.

Its major activity takes place in the central nervous system (in the brain and spinal cord and all they control). But it also sends messages to the peripheral nervous system—all the nervous systems outside the brain and spine—and the peripheral organs, those fed by the peripheral nervous system, importantly including the digestive system.

You're probably seeing where we're going here if you remember the link between the gut and immune function and stress and anxiety, and chronic disease from Chapter 3.

Research shows that plants that affect the endocannabinoid system have the potential for treating a number of disease conditions, including anxiety disorders and neurological disorders like Parkinson's and Huntington's diseases, multiple sclerosis and neuropathic pain plus heart diseases like hardening of the arteries, high blood pressure, stroke and other conditions like glaucoma, metabolic syndrome, osteoporosis and even cancer.

The ECS is also involved in appetite, pain sensation, mood and immune function.

The ECS's almost infinite function shows not only the

widespread networks of receptors, but also enormous possibilities in terms of addressing chronic diseases.

Endocannabinoid receptors and more

The ECS includes a group of endogenous cannabinoid receptors, ligands (molecules that bind one substance to another) and enzymes, molecules that speed up chemical reactions. Receptors, ligands and enzymes are found in virtually every part of the human body.

For some background

Receptors are like little switches on the cell surfaces that, once turned on, cause the cell to act a specific way. For example, an endocannabinoid receptor may be involved with inflammation, so when an endocannabinoid ligand attaches itself to the cell, an anti-inflammatory response occurs. There are ECS receptors associated with nausea, so when these receptors are turned on by endocannabinoid ligands, the end result is nausea relief and so on.

Endocannabinoid ligands bind to the receptors and turn the switches on. What is interesting is that there are molecules in plants that look like endocannabinoid ligands and thus can also impact these switches.

There are two main endocannabinoid receptors, CB1 and CB2. One key ligand called anandamide (the happy and relaxed ligand, its name based on the Sanskrit word for bliss) homes in on those receptors like lasers. Sometimes an imbalance of enzymes knocks anandamide out of circulation, resulting in increased stress and anxiety. See where we're going?

So, now we know that a specialized extract of Echinacea, even at low doses, restores that anandamide balance and keeps you in emotional balance.

It all seems so simple, but we've only known about ECS and ligands and enzymes for a decade or so. Its possibilities are truly life changing for so many people who suffer from unrelieved stress, anxiety disorders and the chronic disease that often results from both. This process is just one example of the ways the ECS receptors, ligands and enzymes can cooperate or fail to cooperate for emotional and physical health and how echinacea can help re-balance when things get wobbly.

Endocannabinoid Deficiency Syndrome

Sometimes shortfalls in key nutrients, especially Omega-3 fatty acids commonly found in fish oil, can also unbalance the ECS, resulting in increased stress and anxiety.

The ECS needs both endocannabinoid compounds and endocannabinoid receptors (think of keys and locks) to properly function. Essential fatty acids, like Omega-3s from fish oil, appear to be the foundation of this combination, making supplementation a key factor in treating anxiety and stress.

> **Your body has the inborn ability to heal itself given the right environment.**

These imbalances can have serious effects. There is scientific evidence that connects ECS deficiency and chronic fatigue syndrome, fibromyalgia, seizure disorders, multiple sclerosis, chronic migraines, irritable bowel syndrome and more.

What causes the ECS deficiency? There are several documented answers, including:

- Omega-3 fatty acid shortfall
- Generally poor diet
- Lifestyle
- Genetic predisposition
- Environmental toxins
- Drug abuse

In 2003, neurologist and psychopharmacologist Ethan Russo, MD, coined the term, "clinical endocannabinoid deficiency syndrome," (CEDS) reflecting the observations seen in clinical research.

CEDS has usually been treated with prescription drugs, which, as we learned earlier, have variable effectiveness and serious side effects.

The concept of improving ECS function opens up a whole new arena of treatment possibilities involving not only stress and anxiety, but many other conditions as well.

Research much like that done with Omega-3s is only scratching the surface of possibilities.

The link between ECS and anxiety

Let's briefly introduce the amygdala, the part of the human brain that detects fear and prepares you for an emergency (fight or flight).

The amygdala consists of two almond-shaped nuclei located deep and medially within the brain in the temporal lobes. From a "bird's eye" view, its location is at the base of the brain.

The amygdala's primary role is to act as a preconscious threat detection system or a central location for the generation of anxiety. It is responsible for the response to emotions such as anger, sadness, and fear as well as the controlling of aggression. Interestingly, the amygdala also retains events and experiences so that you can recognize similar events in the future. Just as in the example in Chapter 6 about a bee sting, the amygdala can store the event, so the next time you see a bee, the memory would increase your anxiety and fear. Put simply, your alertness to a bee would suddenly be increased to help you avoid a bee sting.

The amygdala in humans also is involved in libido or sex drive. According to research conducted by David Reutens at the University of Melbourne, Australia, a man's sex drive may be proportional to the size of his amygdala (not the size of his hands, LOL).

The amygdala has direct connections to the hypothalamus and the brainstem, two areas of the brain related to anxiety and fear. Studies in animals have shown that when the amygdala is removed, the subjects express significantly less fear and anxiety. Human studies show that there is a direct correlation between the activation of the amygdala and the level of anxiety that subjects feel.

At the University of Calgary, endocannabinoid researcher Mathew Hill, Ph.D., made some important observations that can help us better understand the relationship between the amygdala and anxiety. Several studies confirm that people with anxiety disorders often have overactive amygdalas, which may be a major reason for their constant state of anxiety.

Prescription anti-anxiety drugs are designed to slow down the activity of the amygdala.

Now let's connect the amygdala, the ECS receptors and ligands to understand that the endocannabinoid system is a natural regulator of anxiety. Furthermore, endocannabinoid deficiencies may be the cause of anxiety disorders and chronic stress.

Recent animal studies have shown that subjects with genetically low endocannabinoid receptor levels were dramatically anxious and overreacted to stress. They also found that animals with low levels of the ligand anandamide also had high levels of anxiety.

Echinacea

It's been about eight years since the publication of clinical research about *Echinacea angustifolia* and its anti-anxiety effects.

Reporting that the formula is effective within a span of 30 minutes to one hour quite understandably aroused skepticism in the medical community. How could a natural ingredient work that fast?

Most medical practitioners with experience in using a botanical like echinacea say that a quick-acting plant-based medicine that would address anxiety in just a few minutes is questionable, at the least. In fact, until the publication of that pivotal research on echinacea, only prescription drugs like Ativan had that type of claim to fame, along with potentially dire side effects.

Any alternative to highly addictive anxiolytic prescriptions would be very welcome in the world of natural medicine.

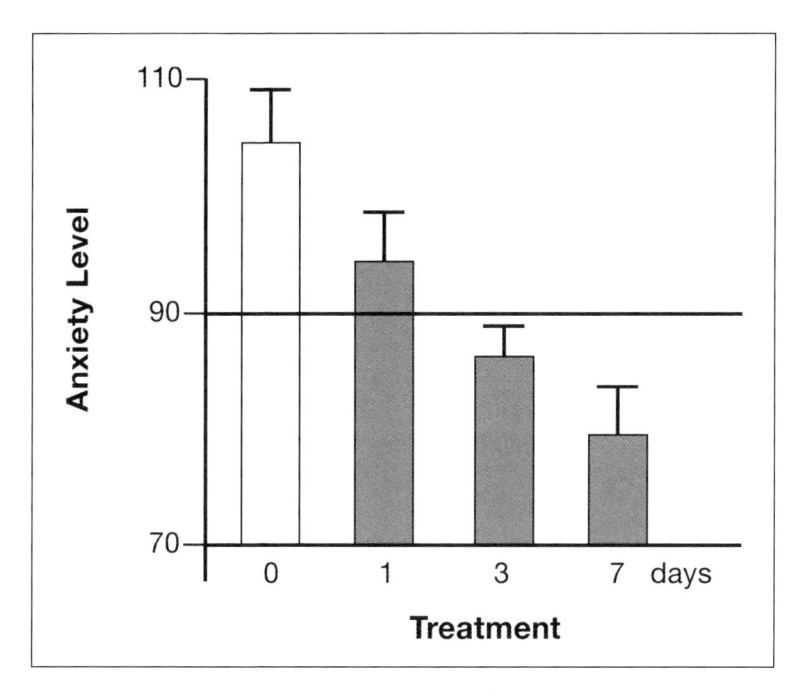

Anxiety levels after treatment with *Echinacea angustifolia*

Josef Haller, Ph.D., head of the department of behavioral neurobiology at the Hungarian Academy of Sciences in Budapest conducted some of the research on *Echinacea angustifolia*. The discovery of this natural medicine came about while Dr. Haller and his team were analyzing a variety of species of Echinacea. Their findings were surprising: Some of the plants contained compounds that could influence brain chemistry, including endocannabinoid receptors.

Of course, echinacea is well-known and has long been studied for the treatment of common colds and flu and it's sometimes used as an anti-inflammatory. The effect is likely due to its ability to rev up the immune system and banish the viruses that cause colds and flu. But the idea that it could have effects on brain chemistry in any way was astonishing.

So, what's happening when a little bit of echinacea can stop a panic attack in its tracks?

An interesting Austrian paper published in 2005 explains how researchers ventured into the realm of anti-anxiety properties of echinacea by looking at its immune-stimulating ability and finding that there is a specific link to the ECS receptors on immune cells, and then normalizing anandamide ligand levels.

This simple observation and some earlier research suggested that a specific extract of this specialized echinacea would have an effect on anxiety.

Getting the right echinacea

To get a better understanding, scientists began comparing a number of species of echinacea plants for the active ingredient that imparted the anti-anxiety effect. Their research found only one species of echinacea—*Echinacea angustifolia*—provided high enough levels of the anxiety-reducing compounds in the proper ratios to effectively reduce anxiety.

In a further follow-up study, seven types of echinacea extracts were compared to the prescription anti-anxiety drug, chlordiazepoxide (a benzodiazepine, Librium is one brand name). Two echinacea preparations showed some mild effects, but only one—from *Echinacea angustifolia*—demonstrated a strong ability to reduce anxiety comparable to the prescription drug.

This special Echinacea root extract not only met the prescription drug's anti-anxiety effects, it exceeded them. It didn't cause any drowsiness—a common side effect of prescription drugs for anxiety. Aside from drowsiness and lethargy, the other side effects of Librium include confusion, edema, nausea, constipation, menstrual abnormalities, jaundice, altered sex drive, involuntary movements, and controlled substance dependence/addiction. None of these negative effects were noted when taking this special extract of echinacea.

What's really important to note here is that a regular echinacea product off the shelf is not going to impart an-ti-anxiety effects. You need to get a specialized extract of echinacea that contains the correct amounts of alkamides, plant compounds that have a variety of benefits, in the proper ratio to relieve anxiety. As far as we have been able to discover, only a specific echinacea extract fits that description.

Human research

In reviewing the clinical research, there is little doubt that *Echinacea angustifolia* works.

- In one study, a 20 mg tablet form was tested on individuals experiencing increased anxiety and tension. After just one day, participants noticed a reduction in stress and anxiety, with a 25% reduction in 7 days.

- In another study published in *Phytotherapy Research* (2012), participants recorded noticeably reduced stress and anxiety in just three days. The study included 33 volunteers (22 women and 11 men) with an average age of 41. All participants were experiencing mild anxiety, assessed using the State-Trait Anxiety Inventory (STAI), a well-accepted method for measuring anxiety levels. In this study, only individuals meeting the threshold for serious anxiety were included in the study. The subjects' anxiety levels were evaluated before, during and after using the specialized echinacea extract for one week. Outcomes showed decreased STAI scores within three days, an effect that remained stable for the duration of the treatment (seven days) and for the two weeks that followed treatment. There were no dropouts and no side effects reported.

- A multi-center, placebo-controlled, double-blind Phase II study involved 26 volunteers and stronger dosage levels. Individuals in the study were diagnosed with generalized anxiety disorder

(GAD) according to DSM-IV (Diagnostics and Statistical Manual of Mental Disorders) criteria. The study started with a screening phase, followed by the six weeks of double-blind treatment. During treatment, participants received either 40 mg of the specialized form of *Echinacea angustifolia* twice daily or placebo tablets twice a day. Between visits one and six during the treatment period, the number of severely anxious patients decreased from 11 to zero in the echinacea group. So, this specialized echinacea preparation significantly reduced anxiety in general anxiety disorder patients, with a full effect within about 21 days.

What is remarkable about this special extract of echinacea is that it has measurable outcomes for subjects with general anxiety disorder. In comparison with anti-anxiety prescription medications, it's a huge bonus that this formula works just as quickly, but with no side effects. The only drugs that work quicker are the benzos, which are accompanied by significant side effects including addiction disorders. This specialized extract of echinacea is free of these side effects, so it's extremely safe on all levels.

Looking to the future with Echinacea

This breakthrough echinacea extract with its unique alkamide composition is just a glimpse into an untapped arena of therapeutic potential.

Since we know the ECS has such a far-reaching role in human body function, it stands to reason that supporting this system and bringing it back into balance can create numerous beneficial health effects. As we continue to explore the world of the ECS and its complexities, it is not difficult to see how this system can become a major asset in improving overall general health, and this unique echinacea formula is the key to safe and effective relief from unrelieved stress and even clinically diagnosed anxiety.

CHAPTER 8

Putting It All Together

From Terry Lemerond

This book has taken us on a journey into the realm of stress and anxiety and revealed the serious life-disrupting effects of anxiety when it becomes all-consuming. The goal was to attain a better understanding about these health consequences and alternative options to halt the downward spiral.

As promised, we've discussed a truly powerful option: a specialized extract of *Echinacea angustifolia*. Unlike any other botanical we know, with most people, this extract of echinacea is fast acting, safe and effective. It offers a useful new tool for people with anxiety disorders and a broad-ranging solution for numerous other conditions resulting from unrelieved stress.

This unique echinacea extract, with its active compounds known as alkamides, works by impacting specific endocannabinoid receptors resulting in impressive anxiety calming effects.

Many people are not comfortable taking prescription drugs for stress, anxiety and insomnia. Interestingly, in addition to their negative side effects, many of these drugs work well for a short period of time, but as the body develops tolerance over time, they become frustratingly less effective.

If you are taking prescription drugs for anxiety, stress or insomnia and you want to stop taking them, I cannot emphasize strongly enough, that you *must* consult your doctor and make a structured plan for coming off them gradually. These drugs are highly addictive if you have taken them for more than four weeks (that's right, *four* weeks!).

Withdrawal, if done "cold turkey" can be extremely unpleasant and have serious consequential effects. Again, make sure you consult your physician or a health care provider who can give you professional guidance.

If you know you are suffering from the effects of prolonged stress and anxiety, and especially if you have been diagnosed with an anxiety disorder, I highly recommend you try *Echinacea angustifolia*.

If you and your health care provider have decided to wean yourself from pharmaceuticals in favor of side-effect free and non-addictive echinacea, make your plan together to minimize the withdrawal effects.

Either way, here are some steps that can help make your transition easier.

Step 1: First Action

Every treatment plan needs a foundational component. When it comes to stress and anxiety, a specialized extract of echinacea should get top consideration.

If you are not taking prescription anxiety/stress medication, take two tablets twice daily for the first week and then reduce to 2 tablets daily. Eventually, you'll be able to take this only when you need it.

If you are on prescription medications for anxiety/stress, you can take this echinacea, but as I mentioned earlier you must consult with your family doctor or prescribing physician.

Most people get relief from an anxiety episode in as little as 30 to 60 minutes by taking two tablets, although there are those that can feel relief even sooner. Some people start seeing results in their general susceptibility to anxiety issues and a substantial reduction in the number of anxiety events after four to five days by taking two tablets a day.

Some practitioners have reported positive results to me that they have given the formula to children as young as 4 years of age at the dosage of one tablet daily.

This clinically studied echinacea is quite effective for insomnia. Two tablets at bedtime can help you sleep, especially if your insomnia is the result of chronic stress and anxiety.

This product is extremely safe, has no addictive properties and can be used with confidence.

Step 2: Adrenal Support

As we've mentioned, the adrenal glands are an important line of defense to any type of stress and anxiety. They produce hormones that help the body control blood sugar, break down protein and fat, react to stressors like a major illness or injury, and regulate blood pressure. Cortisol and aldosterone, adrenaline and sex hormones called androgens are the most important adrenal hormones.

As you'll recall from Chapter 4, long-term exposure to stress and anxiety can cause the adrenals to become overused, fatigued and eventually create adrenal exhaustion. Adrenal support to prevent overuse, fatigue and exhaustion is an important step in overall treatment of stress and anxiety and involves two actions:

1. Get good quality protein in your regimen: I recommend one gram of protein per pound of body weight, so if you weigh 150 pounds, you should eat 150 grams of protein a day.

2. Take an adrenal support formula as mentioned in Chapter 4. Take 1 or 2 capsules of a high-quality product either with breakfast or lunch to avoid any issues with sleep.

Final Comments

As we've mentioned several times, your body has an innate ability to heal itself if you provide the right environment. We've discussed numerous tools to make that happen and introduced you to a powerful solution, the special formulation of the familiar herb used to treat colds and flu, *Echinacea angustifolia*. The specialized extract of echinacea can help you reduce anxiety and stress quickly and without consequential side effects.

Most of us are aware on some level that unrelieved stress and anxiety are underlying causes of numerous chronic diseases. In Chapter 3, you learned about the one-cell deep intestinal lining and how chronic stress can lead to a dysfunctional immune system, through a series of events creating "leaky gut."

In Chapter 4, we took a look at the adrenal glands and the importance they play in stress and anxiety. The adrenal hormones are vital components of controlling the stress response and controlling blood sugar, blood pressure and other body needs during demanding conditions. When stress and anxiety become prolonged, the adrenal glands can become compromised creating further health issues.

In Chapter 6, we gave you a list of nutritional and botanical compounds with scientific research proven to support stress and anxiety relief.

And in Chapter 7, we took a deep look at the newly discovered and all-important endocannabinoid system (ECS) and how the specialized extract of *Echinacea angustifolia* impacts the ECS and thus helps reduce the feelings of anxiety.

I am beyond impressed with the results that have been reported to me by medical professionals who have used this breakthrough treatment for several years now.

CHAPTER 9

Doc to Doc

From Dr. Wagner

Dear Doctor,

Like most books, this book is copyrighted. However, the information presented here is so important to your patients' health as well as to your scientific knowledge, we have urged our readers to copy this chapter and give it to you. My hope is that this summary of efficacy of a specific formulation of *Echinacea angustifolia* will help you recognize its effectiveness and value to your patients. I have seen it treat depression and anxiety and even to relieve acute anxiety within minutes.

First, let me briefly introduce myself:

I am Lynn Wagner, MD, an integrative medicine physician. Early in my medical career as an emergency medicine physician, I saw unnecessary disease and suffering, often the result of lives lived out of balance. I decided to study the field of integrative medicine, a specialty that uses both conventional and non-conventional medicine to help patients reach their health goals. I now use my integrative training as the foundation of my private practice.

When I learned about this unique formulation of *Echinacea angustifolia* and saw the impressive results among my patients, I knew that its anti-anxiolytic properties must be shared with my colleagues.

Unlike any other botanical I've encountered, this extract can offer relief for an acute anxiety episode within 30 minutes or less.

Clinical studies show that longer term and regular use of the echinacea product reduce the incidence of acute anxiety, improve resiliency in the face of chronic stress and improve quality of life in people with mild to moderate depression.

You are certainly aware of various pharmaceuticals that address chronic stress, depression, and anxiety. You are also fully aware of the potential for disastrous side effects of many drugs, especially benzodiazepines.

I've found a specific extract of *Echinacea angustifolia* to be a safe and efficacious alternative.

For most of us who have ventured into the world of botanical healing, echinacea is well-known as an immunoenhancer. You may also be aware that immune health and gut health support neurotransmitter health, especially through the production of dopamine and serotonin.

Enhanced immune function and gut health can lead to increased resiliency in the face of chronic stress along with a reduction in the anxiety and insomnia that comes along with that stress. This is the foundation for how *Echinacea angustifolia* works.

How exactly does *Echinacea angustifolia* actually do this?

Through the endocannabinoid system (ECS).

In a comparison test of seven different echinacea extracts, only one—*Echinacea angustifolia* root—was able to activate the body's ECS and stimulate neurotransmitter production, which effectively provides relief from acute and chronic anxiety.

The ECS contains two main endocannabinoid receptors, CB1 and CB2. There is a key ligand called anandamide that is our body's natural cannabinoid. It attaches to these receptors strongly. Sometimes an enzymatic imbalance suppresses anandamide production, resulting in increased stress and anxiety. This specialized extract of echinacea, even at low doses, can restore that anandamide balance.

Balance in the ECS goes far beyond mental health. The ECS is also involved in appetite, pain sensation, mood and immune function. Research suggests that plants that affect the endocannabinoid system have the potential for treating a number of disease conditions, not just anxiety disorders. They can help diseases like neurological disorders (Parkinson's and Huntington's diseases), multiple sclerosis and neuropathic pain. They can improve inflammatory conditions like atherosclerosis, hypertension, ischemic stroke, metabolic syndrome and osteoporosis. There is research suggesting they can help conditions like glaucoma and even some types of cancer.

What makes this formulation different from other echinacea?

Researchers at the Hungarian Academy of Sciences found that some echinacea plants contained compounds known to influence brain chemistry and greatly reduce anxiety. Further exploration revealed that it is not just the species of echinacea that is important, but the cultivation and extraction process that makes it unique.

Clinical trials confirmed mental health benefits of *Echinacea angustifolia*. In subjects who reported experiencing *increased* stress and tension, a standardized anxiety assessment was used to measure their feelings of anxiety at the beginning of the study and compared with responses 1, 3, and 7 days after taking the specialized extract. After one day of use, the participants experienced a significant reduction on the anxiety measurement scale, which increased to a 25% reduction by Day 7.

Better yet, the results did not cause drowsiness, a common side effect of prescription anti-anxiety drugs or any other side effects.

In reviewing the clinical research, there is little doubt that *Echinacea angustifolia* works:

- In one study, a 20 mg tablet form was tested on individuals experiencing increased anxiety and tension. After just one day, participants noticed a reduction in stress and anxiety, with a 25% reduction in 7 days.

- In another study published in *Phytotherapy Research* (2012), participants recorded noticeably reduced stress and anxiety in just three days. The study included 33 volunteers (22 women and 11 men) with an average age of 41. All participants were experiencing mild anxiety, assessed using the State-Trait Anxiety Inventory (STAI), a well-accepted method for measuring anxiety levels. In this study, only individuals meeting the threshold for serious anxiety were included in the study. The subjects' anxiety levels were evaluated before, during and after using the specialized echinacea extract for one week. Outcomes showed decreased STAI scores within three days, an effect that remained stable for the duration of the treatment (seven days) and for the two weeks that followed treatment. There were no dropouts and no side effects reported.

- A multi-center, placebo-controlled, double-blind Phase II study involved 26 volunteers and stronger dosage levels. Individuals in the study were diagnosed with generalized anxiety disorder (GAD) according to DSM-IV. The study started with a screening phase, followed by the six weeks of double-blind treatment. During treatment, participants received either 40 mg of the specialized form of *Echinacea angustifolia* twice daily or placebo tablets twice a day. Between visits one and six during the treatment period, the number of severely anxious patients decreased from 11 to zero in the echinacea group. So, this specialized echinacea preparation significantly reduced anxiety in general anxiety disorder patients, with a full effect within about 21 days.

- A 2012 Hungarian clinical trial confirmed that the echinacea preparation was as effective as the benzodiazepine chlordiazepoxide (Librium) without side effects.

- An interesting Austrian paper published in 2005 explains how researchers ventured into the realm of anti-anxiety properties of echinacea by looking at its immune-stimulating ability and finding that there is a specific link to the ECS receptors on immune cells, and then normalizing anandamide ligand levels.

Echinacea angustifolia is my choice as a safe and natural alternative for those suffering from stress and its effects. I encourage you to try it with your patients and experience the anxiety and stress relief I have seen in mine.

—*Lynn Wagner, M.D.*

References

Haller J, Krecsak et al. Double-blind placebo-controlled trial of the anxiolytic effects of a standardized Echinacea extract. *Phytother Res.* 2020 Mar;34(3):660–668.

Haller J, Freund TF, Pelczer KG, et al. The anxiolytic potential and psychotropic side effects of an Echinacea preparation in laboratory animals and healthy volunteers. *Phytotherapy Research.* 2013: Jan;27(1):54–61

Haller J, Hohmann J, Freund TF. The effect of Echinacea preparations in three laboratory tests of anxiety: comparison with chlordiazepoxide. *Phytother Res.* 2010 Nov;24(11):1605–13

Holmes TH, Rahe RH. The social readjustment rating scale. *J Psychosom Res* 1967;11:213–218.

Törnhage CJ. Salivary cortisol for assessment of hypothalamic-pituitary-adrenal axis function. *Neuroimmunomodulation.* 2009;16(5):284–9.

Stetler C, Miller GE. Blunted cortisol response to awakening in mild to moderate depression: regulatory influences of sleep patterns and social contacts. *J Abnorm Psychol.* 2005 Nov;114(4):697–705.

Mallon L, Broman JE, Hetta J. Is usage of hypnotics associated with mortality? *Sleep Med.* 2009 Mar;10(3):279–86.

Wyatt RJ. The serotonin-catecholamine-dream bicycle. A clinical study. *Biol Psychiatry* 1972;5:33–64.

Guilleminault C, Cathala HP, Castaigne P. Effects of 5-HTP on sleep of a patient with brain stem lesion. *Electroencephalogr Clin Neurophysiol* 1973;34:177–184.

Wyatt RJ, Zarcone V, Engelman K. Effects of 5-hydroxytryptophan on the sleep of normal human subjects. *Electroencephalogr Clin Neurophysiol* 1971;30:505–509.

Autret A, Minz M, Bussel B, et al. Human sleep and 5-HTP. Effects of repeated high doses and of association with benserazide. *Electroencephalogr Clin Neurophysiol* 1976;41:408–413.

Soulairac A, Lambinet H. Effect of 5-hydroxytryptophan, a serotonin precursor, on sleep disorders. *Ann Med Psychol* (Paris) 1977;1:792–798.

Eschenauer G, Sweet BV. Pharmacology and therapeutic uses of theanine. *Am J Health Syst Pharm*. 2006;63(1):26, 28–30.

Vuksan V, Sievenpiper JL, Owen R, et al. Beneficial effects of viscous dietary fiber from Konjac-mannan in subjects with the insulin resistance syndrome: results of a controlled metabolic trial. *Diabetes Care* 2000;23:9–14.

Freeman MP, Rapaport MH. Omega-3 fatty acids and depression: from cellular mechanisms to clinical care. *J Clin Psychiatry*. 2011 Feb;72(2):258–9.

Buydens-Branchey L, Branchey M, Hibbeln JR. Associations between increases in plasma n-3 polyunsaturated fatty acids following supplementation and decreases in anger and anxiety in substance abusers. *Prog Neuropsychopharmacol Biol Psychiatry* 2008;32:568–575.

Möller HJ. Is there evidence for negative effects of antidepressants on suicidality in depressive patients? A systematic review. *Eur Arch Psychiatry Clin Neurosci*. 2006 Dec;256(8):476–96.

Rudin DO. The major psychoses and neuroses as omega-3 essential fatty acid deficiency syndrome: substrate pellagra. *Biol Psychiatry* 1981;16:837–50.

Moncrieff J, Cohen D. Do antidepressants cure or create abnormal brain states? *PLoS Med*. 2006 Jul;3(7):e240.

Middleton H, Moncrieff J. 'They won't do any harm and might do some good': time to think again on the use of antidepressants? *Br J Gen Pract*. 2011 Jan;61(582):47–9

Fournier JC, DeRubeis RJ, Hollon SD, Dimidjian S, Amsterdam JD, Shelton RC, Fawcett J. Antidepressant drug effects and depression severity: a patient-level meta-analysis. *JAMA*. 2010;303(1):47–53.

Byerley WF, Judd LL, Reimherr FW, et al. 5-Hydroxytryptophan: a review of its antidepressant efficacy and adverse effects. *J Clin Psychopharmacol* 1987;7:127–137.

Gilliland K, Bullock W. Caffeine: a potential drug of abuse. *Adv Alcohol Subst Abuse* 1984;3:53–73.

Greden J, Fontaine P, Lubetsky M, et al. Anxiety and depression associated with caffeinism among psychiatric inpatients. *Am J Psychiatry* 1978;135:963–966.

Neil JF, Himmelhoch JM, Mallinger AG, et al. Caffeinism complicating hypersomnic depressive episodes. *Compr Psychiatry* 1978;19: 377–385.

Charney D, Heninger G, Jatlow P. Increased anxiogenic effects of caffeine in panic disorders. *Arch Gen Psychiatry* 1985;42:233–243.

Kreitsch K. Prevalence, presenting symptoms, and psychological characteristics of individuals experiencing a diet-related mood disturbance. *Behav Ther* 1985;19:593–594.

Christensen L. Psychological distress and diet—effects of sucrose and caffeine. *J Appl Nutr* 1988;40:44–50.

Abdoua AM, Higashiguchia S, Horiea K, et al. Relaxation and immunity enhancement effects of Gamma-Aminobutyric acid (GABA) administration in humans. *BioFactors* 2006;26:201–208

Shevtsov VA, Zholus BI, Shervarly VI, et al. A randomized trial of two different doses of a SHR-5 Rhodiola rosea extract versus placebo and control of capacity for mental work. *Phytomedicine* 2003;10:95–105.

Darbinyan V, Kteyan A, Panossian A, et al. Rhodiola rosea in stress induced fatigue—a double blind cross-over study of a standardized extract SHR-5 with a repeated low-dose regimen on the mental performance of healthy physicians during night duty. *Phytomedicine* 2000;7:365–371.

Spasov AA, Wikman GK, Mandrikov VB, et al. A double-blind, placebo-controlled pilot study of the stimulating and adaptogenic effect of Rhodiola rosea SHR-5 extract on the fatigue of students caused by stress during an examination period with a repeated low-dose regimen. *Phytomedicine* 2000;7:85–89.

Olsson EM, von Schéele B, Panossian AG. A randomised, double-blind, placebo-controlled, parallel-group study of the standardised extract shr-5 of the roots of Rhodiola rosea in the treatment of subjects with stress-related fatigue. *Planta Med.* 2009 Feb;75(2):105–12.

Auddy B, Hazra J, Mitra A, Abedon B, Ghosal S. A standardized Withania somnifera extract significantly reduces stress-related parameters in chronically stressed humans: a double-blind, randomized, placebo-controlled study. *JANA* 2008;11:50–6

Akhondzadeh S, Kashani L, Fotouhi A, et al. Comparison of Lavandula angustifolia Mill. tincture and imipramine in the treatment of mild to moderate depression: a double-blind, randomized trial. *Prog Neuropsychopharmacol Biol Psychiatry.* 2003;27:123–7.

Baird AD, Wilson SJ, Bladin PF, et al. The amygdala and sexual drive: insights from temporal lobe epilepsy surgery. *Ann Neurology.* 2004; Jan: 55(1):87–96

Woelkart K, Bauer R. et al. The role of alkamides as an active principle in echinacea. *Planta Medica.* 2007 Jun;73(7): 615–23

Kessler RC, Ruscio AM, Shear K, Wittchen HU. Epidemiology of anxiety disorders. *Curr Top Behav Neurosci.* 2010;2:21–35.

Culpepper L. Generalized anxiety disorder and medical illness. *J Clin Psychiatry.* 2009;70(Suppl 2):20–24

Weisberg RB. Overview of generalized anxiety disorder: epidemiology, presentation, and course. *J Clin Psychiatry.* 2009;70(Suppl 2):4–9.

Cantor C. Post-traumatic stress disorder: evolutionary perspectives. *Aust N Z J Psychiatry.* 2009;43(11):1038–48

Tolin DF. Is cognitive-behavioral therapy more effective than other therapies? A meta-analytic review. *Clin Psychol Rev.* 2010;30(6):710–20.

Durant C, Christmas D, Nutt D. The pharmacology of anxiety. *Curr Top Behav Neurosci.* 2010;2:303–30.

Ruhe HG, Mason NS, Schene AH. Mood is indirectly related to serotonin, norepinephrine and dopamine levels in humans: a meta-analysis of monoamine depletion studies. *Mol Psychiatry.* 2007;12:331–59.

Cloos JM, Ferreira V. Current use of benzodiazepines in anxiety disorders. *Curr Opin Psychiatry.* 2009;22(1):90–95.

Young SN. How to increase serotonin in the human brain without drugs. *J Psychiatry Neurosci.* 2007;32(6):394–99.

Lakhan SE, Vieira KF. Nutritional therapies for mental disorders. *Nutr J.* 2008;7:2.

REFERENCES

Carroll D, Ring C, Suter M, Willemsen G. The effects of an oral multivitamin combination with calcium, magnesium, and zinc on psychological well-being in healthy young male volunteers: a double-blind placebo-controlled trial. *Psychopharmacology* (Berl) 2000;150(2):220–25.

De Souza MC, Walker AF, Robinson PA, Bolland K. A synergistic effect of a daily supplement for 1 month of 200 mg magnesium plus 50 mg vitamin B6 for the relief of anxiety-related premenstrual symptoms: a randomized, double-blind, crossover study. *J Womens Health Gend Based Med*. 2000;9(2):131–39

Appleton KM, Rogers PJ, Ness AR. Is there a role for n-3 long-chain polyunsaturated fatty acids in the regulation of mood and behaviour? A review of the evidence to date from epidemiological studies, clinical studies and intervention trials. *Nutr Res Rev*. 2008;21(1):13–41.

Kiecolt-Glaser JK, Belury MA, Andridge R, et al. Omega-3 supplementation lowers inflammation and anxiety in medical students: a randomized controlled trial. *Brain Behav Immun*. 2011;25(8):1725–34.

Buydens-Branchey L, Branchey M, Hibbeln JR. Associations between increases in plasma n-3 polyunsaturated fatty acids following supplementation and decreases in anger and anxiety in substance abusers. *Prog Neuropsychopharmacol Biol Psychiatry*. 2008;32(2):568–75.

Perica MM, Delas I. Essential Fatty acids and psychiatric disorders. *Nutr Clin Pract*. 2011;26(4):409–25.

Ross BM. Omega-3 polyunsaturated fatty acids and anxiety disorders. *Prostaglandins Leukot Essent Fatty Acids*. 2009;81(5–6):309–12.

Bhattacharya SK, Bhattacharya A, Sairam K, Ghosal S. Anxiolytic-antidepressant activity of Withania somnifera glycowithanolides: an experimental study. *Phytomedicine*. 2000;7(6):463–69.

Kalman DS, Feldman S, Feldman R, et al. Effect of a proprietary Magnolia and Phellodendron extract on stress levels in healthy women: a pilot, double-blind, placebo-controlled clinical trial. *Nutr J*. 2008;7:11.

Kakuda T. Neuroprotective effects of theanine and its preventive effects on cognitive dysfunction. *Pharmacol Res*. 2011;64(2):162–68.

Index

ACTH, 9
adrenal exhaustion. *See* adrenal fatigue
adrenal extracts, 41
adrenal fatigue, 35–37, 59, 79–80
   causes, 38
   symptoms, 36, 39
adrenal glands, 7–8, 10, 35–42, 79–80
   excessive activity of, 37
   support for, 40–42, 79
adrenaline, 10, 35, 38, 79
adrenocorticotropic hormone (ACTH). *See* ACTH
AGES, 58
aldosterone, 35, 42, 79
alkamides, 74, 76, 77
amygdala, 8, 56, 70–71
anandamide, 68, 71, 73, 82, 85
androgens, 79
antiacids, 32
antibodies, 27
antidepressants, 54
anxiety, 5–6, 13–14, 15–24, 71, 82, 84–85
   definition, 15
   diet and, 23, 24, 57–60
   diseases and, 25–34, 79
   normal, 15–16, 17–18
   questionnaire on, 24
   symptoms, 15–16
anxiety disorders, 16, 18–24, 71
   causes, 22
   depression and, 19, 21, 24, 54
   diagnosis of, 21
   symptoms, 21
   treatment, 22–23
   treatment (botanical/nutritional), 23, 60–62, 63, 64–65, 72–76, 80
   treatment (pharmaceutical), 22, 53–55, 77–78
   types, 18–20
Ativan, 22, 72

bacteria, 27, 29–30
benzodiazepines, 53–55, 73–74, 75
blood pressure, 8, 10, 36, 37
blood sugar. *See* glucose
brain, 22, 54, 55, 56, 64, 70, 73
brainstem, 71
breathing
   belly/diaphragmatic, 47–49

C. difficile, 29–30
caffeine, 58–60
cancers, 3
cardiovascular disease, 3
CBT. *See* cognitive behavior therapy (CBT)

CEDS. *See* clinical endocannabinoid deficiency syndrome (CEDS)
cells, 4–5, 58
  barrier, 30–34
  epithelial, 30–34
  nerve, 22
cholesterol, 37
chronic obstructive pulmonary disorder (COPD). *See* COPD
clinical endocannabinoid deficiency syndrome (CEDS), 70
coffee. *See* caffeine
cognitive behavior therapy (CBT), 43–45
compulsions, 20
COPD, 25
coping strategies, 22–23, 43–52
Cordain, Loren, 40–41
cortisol, 10, 35, 37, 38–39, 42, 59, 79

depression, 19, 21, 24, 54
dehydroepiandrosterone (DHEA). *See* DHEA
DHEA, 42
diabetes, 58
  Type 2, 4
diet, 23, 24, 57–60
digestive system. *See* gut
diseases, 13
diseases (chronic), 4, 25–34, 68, 79
  gut permeability and, 31–34
  stress and, 11, 12, 25–34, 67, 79

echinacea, 50, 60, 63, 73, 84

Echinacea angustifolia, 60, 63–65, 72–76, 77, 78–79, 80, 81–85
ECS. *See* endocannabinoid system (ECS)
EFAs. *See* essential fatty acids (EFAs)
EFT, 47
EMDR, 47
emotional freedom technique (EFT). *See* EFT
emotions, 56, 71
endocannabinoid deficiency syndrome. *See* clinical endocannabinoid deficiency syndrome (CEDS)
endocannabinoid system (ECS), 42, 65–71, 76, 80, 82–83
endocannabinoids, 66, 82
endorphins, 45
energy (cellular), 4–5, 10
energy drinks, 59
enzymes
  endocannabinoid, 68–69, 82
epinephrine, 59
essential fatty acids (EFAs), 69
exercise, 45–46
eye movement desensitization and processing (EMDR). *See* EMDR

fat (abdominal), 39
fear, 15, 19–20
fecal transplantation, 29
fight or flight response, 7–8, 16, 32
fish oil, 69

GABA, 54, 56, 59

GAD. *See* generalized anxiety disorder (GAD)
gamma-aminobutyric acid (GABA). *See* GABA
GAS. *See* general adaptation syndrome (GAS)
gastrointestinal tract. *See* gut
general adaptation syndrome (GAS), 9–13
   alarm reaction, 9–10
   exhaustion stage, 11–13
   resistance phase, 10–11
generalized anxiety disorder (GAD), 18, 22, 75, 85
genetics, 22, 25
glucose, 8, 10, 36, 37, 38, 59
glycation, 58
glycogen, 10, 37
gut, 26–34, 67
   bacteria in, 27, 29–30
   disorders, 25
   exposure to external environment, 27–28
   immune system and, 26, 27–28, 80
   lining of, 11, 30–34, 80
   neurotransmitters and, 28–29
   permeability of, 30–34, 80

Haller, Josef, 72–73
heart attacks, 11, 21, 25
Hill, Matthew, 71
Hippocrates, 26
hops, 60
HPA axis, 56
human body, 51–52, 66–68
   self-healing of, 51–52, 62, 80
Hungarian Academy of Sciences, 64, 74, 83–84
hypnosis, 47
hypothalamus, 9, 32, 38, 71
hypothalamus-pituitary-adrenal axis. *See* HPA axis

IgG, 27
immune system, 26, 27–28, 39, 63, 73, 82, 85
immunoglobulin G. *See* IgG
inflammation, 38–39

lavender, 60
leaky gut. *See* gut: permeability of
Librium, 73–74, 87
lifestyle, 23, 24, 25, 40, 51–52
ligands
   endocannabinoid, 68, 71, 73, 82, 85
lorazepam. *See* Ativan
L-tyrosine, 41

marijuana, 66
memory, 56, 71
microbiome, 27, 29–30
mitochondria, 4–5

nature, 45–46
nervous system, 54, 67
   sympathetic, 7, 32–33
neurotransmitters, 28–29, 56, 59, 82
nutraceuticals. *See* supplements

obsessions, 20
obsessive-compulsive disorder (OCD), 20
OCD. *See* obsessive-compulsive disorder (OCD)
omega-3 fatty acids, 69

one cell paradox, 30–34, 80
oxidative stress, 5

panic attacks. *See* panic disorder
panic disorder, 18–19
pantothenic acid. *See* vitamin B5
personality, 25
phobias, 19–20
pituitary gland, 9
plaque
   arterial, 26
post-traumatic stress disorder (PTSD), 20–21
prednisone, 38–39
pregnenolone, 42
progesterone, 42
protein, 40–41, 80
PTSD. *See* post-traumatic stress disorder (PTSD)
pyridoxal-5-phosphate, *See* vitamin B6
receptors, 66
   endocannabinoid, 66, 68–69, 71, 73, 77, 82
relaxation, 46
Reutens, David, 71
Russo, Ethan, 70

salt, 36
selective serotonin uptake inhibitors (SSRIs). *See* SSRIs
Selye, Hans, 9
serotonin, 28–29, 54
sex drive, 71
sleep, 49–50, 59, 60, 79
social anxiety disorder, 19
sodas, 59
SSRIs, 28–29, 54

STAI. *See* State-Trait Anxiety Inventory (STAI)
startle responses, 17–18
State-Trait Anxiety Inventory (STAI), 75, 84
stevia, 60
stomach acid, 26
stress, 6–13, 71
   chronic, 9, 12–13, 39, 82
   diet and, 57–60
   diseases and, 7, 11, 12–13, 25–34, 39, 79
   management of, 9, 43–52
stressors, 10, 11–12
strokes, 11
sugar, 57–58, 60
supplements, 23, 24, 60–62
   for adrenal support, 40, 41–42
sweeteners, 57
swimming, 45

tea, 59, 60
thoughts
   negative, 44, 45
tight junctions, 31
traumas, 20

valerian, 60
vitamin B5, 41
vitamin B6, 41

walking, 45
weight, 39
Wilson, James, 36

Zebra and Lion story, 7–8, 14, 32–33, 35–36

About the Authors

Lynn Wagner, MD

Dr. Lynn Wagner believes that true healing starts with a healthy lifestyle, incorporates healing modalities from both traditional and non-traditional medicine and looks at the patient's entire health story. Early in her career as an emergency medicine physician, she saw unnecessary disease and suffering, often the result of a life lived out of balance. By incorporating principles of integrative medicine, into her practice, a specialty that utilizes lifestyle and traditional and non-traditional medical practices, she is able to help her patients achieve their health goals by taking control over their personal health and getting back into balance.

Terry Lemerond

Terry Lemerond is a natural health expert with over 55 years of experience. He has owned health food stores, founded dietary supplement companies, and formulated over 500 products. A much sought-after speaker and accomplished author, Terry shares his wealth of experience and knowledge in health and nutrition through his educational programs, including the *Terry Talks Nutrition* website (https://www.terrytalksnutrition.com), newsletters, podcasts, webinars, and personal speaking engagements. His books include *Seven Keys to Vibrant Health* and the sequel, *Seven Keys to Unlimited Personal Achievement,* and his newest publication, *50+ Natural Health Secrets Proven to Change Your Life.* His continual dedication, energy, and zeal are part of his ongoing mission to improve the health of America.